HEALING HOUSEPLANTS

HOW TO KEEP PLANTS INDOORS FOR CLEAN AIR, HEALTHIER SKIN, IMPROVED FOCUS, AND A HAPPIER LIFE!

MICHELLE POLK

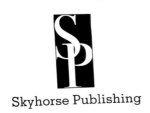

Skyhorse Publishing

Skyhorse Publishing books may be purchased in bulk at special discounts for sales promotion, corporate gifts, fund-raising, or educational purposes. Special editions can also be created to specifications. For details, contact the Special Sales Department, Skyhorse Publishing, 307 West 36th Street, 11th Floor, New York, NY 10018 or info@ skyhorsepublishing.com.

Skyhorse® and Skyhorse Publishing® are registered trademarks of Skyhorse Publishing, Inc.®, a Delaware corporation.

Visit our website at www.skyhorsepublishing.com.

10 9 8 7 6 5 4 3 2 1

Library of Congress Cataloging-in-Publication Data is available on file.

Cover design by Mona Lin
Cover image courtesy of iStock.com

Print ISBN: 978-1-51073-132-5
Ebook ISBN: 978-1-51073-133-2

Printed in China

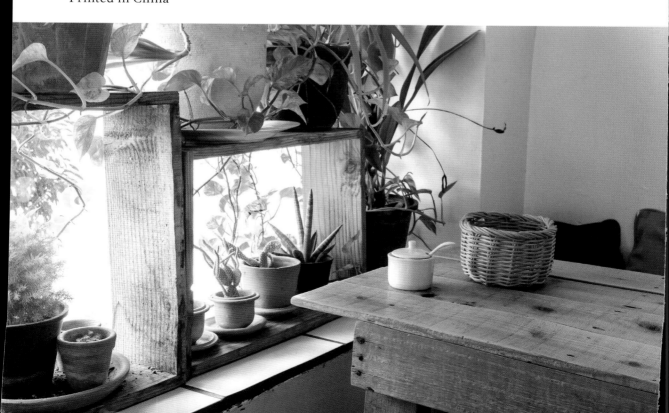

Contents

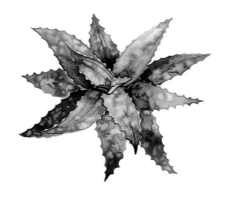

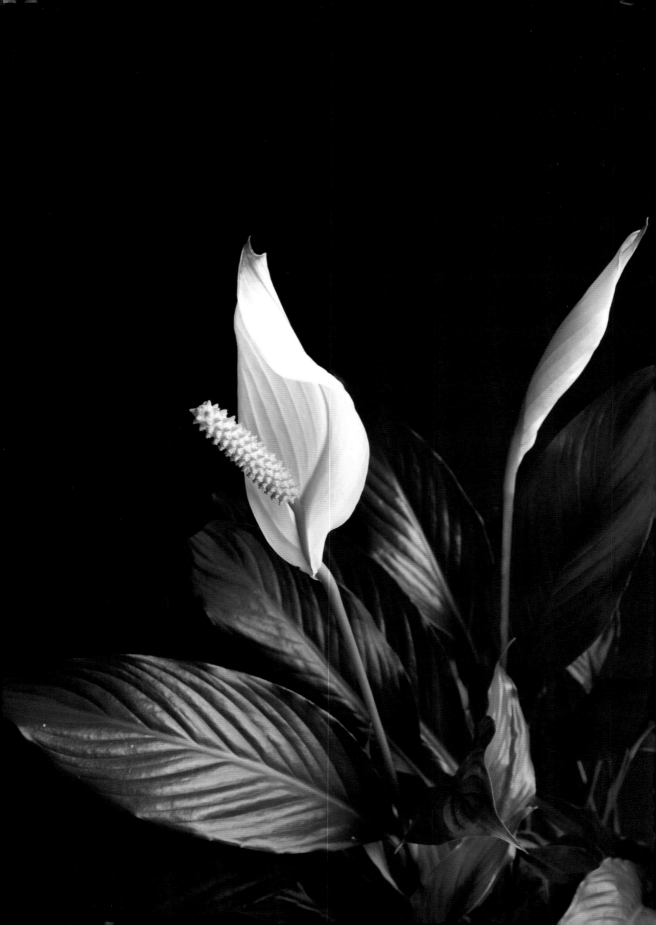

Preface

Herbs and plants are some of the most amazing inhabitants of our planet; beautiful, complicated, mysterious, and extremely beneficial to humans, plants also keep us alive. And while this book is dedicated to the immense healing benefits of plants for our health and well-being, I would be remiss to say they were all beneficial and safe.

Plants have evolved with self-defense mechanisms, many of which can be turned into healing properties for humans, saving us from infections, chronic illnesses, cancers, and more. However, that is not to say that all plants are harmless bystanders, growing in dirt, just waiting to help us heal.

Many plants are extremely dangerous, not only to humans but to our pets as well, posing immense threats and danger if consumed, ingested, or even simply exposed to our skin. Just think of poison ivy. While it's not life-threatening, no one wishes to be scathed by this annoying plant.

You might be nodding in agreement with these statements, but many people don't realize how dangerous some innocent-seeming herbs can be to a certain percentage of the population. Plants like lavender, rosemary, mint, or aloe can be dangerous if given to the right person at the wrong time, or while they are taking the wrong medication.

I strongly urge you to consult your doctor or health care practitioner before consuming herbs or plants, especially if you're taking certain medications. The pharmaceutical cocktails many people are currently on can make you more susceptible to reactions from plants and herbs, and you can never be too safe. While growing lavender in your home is perfectly innocuous, don't be the one person who is sent to the hospital due to an interaction with a drug or prescription medication.

Even the most innocent plants are deadly at the right doses. So do yourself a favor and do your homework.

Outlined in the chapters to follow is a section dedicated to warnings, precautions, and possible interactions with drugs. Some of the information may seem scary, where everything may appear deadly. However, even water, at the right dose, is deadly, so don't be fearful when you see warnings for even the most innocuous-seeming plants, like mint. Just be cautious.

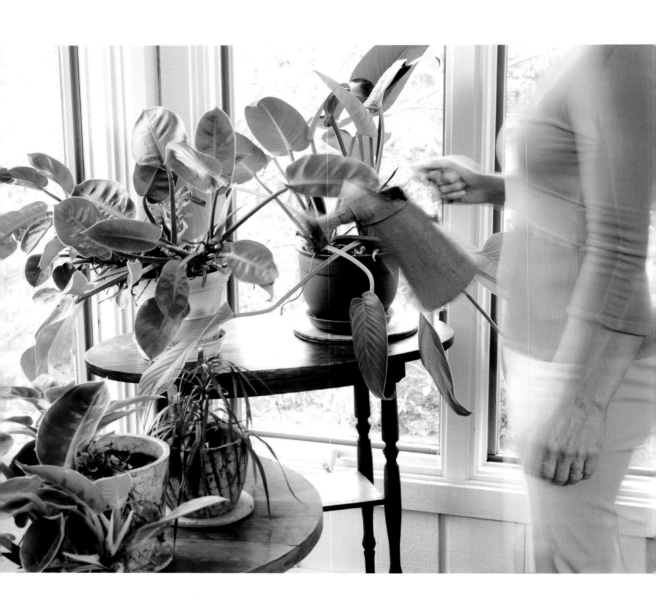

Introduction

I grew up in a home surrounded by plants; green leaves were as much a fixture of the decor as the painted walls. Ferns would drape their long fronds over furniture, lemon trees made a point of confusing my little mind as they thrived in the Chicago winter months, and jade plants would regenerate their thick green leaves into offspring on every nook and cranny in every room in the house.

My mother has what you would call a green thumb. Her gardening skills flourished in our house and backyard, creating an ambiance resembling sunny Miami rather than frigid Chicago. My mom's mantra in the summers was, "Please, take more tomatoes, I've grown way too many!" Our backyard resembled a jungle rather than a suburban patio, and we got to enjoy every bright hydrangea, juicy tomato, colorful tulip, and spicy pepper she cultivated.

So it came as quite a surprise when I killed my first dozen plants after leaving for college. *There must be something wrong,* I thought. I was the daughter of the best gardener I knew. I must have picked up some knowledge throughout the years, or at least have some sort of innate green thumb waiting to sprout up, right? I never imagined how truly horrible a gardener I could be. I killed more plants in the next few years than I could count. I overwatered, undernourished, overfed, underwatered, and burned dozens of plants. And these incidents didn't include the carnage caused by my cat.

I became so inept at caring for plants that I thought I was cursed. It came to the point where my mom stopped gifting me her extra jade plants and solely handed them out to my brother—that's some real plant shame.

Fast forward several years, and I became fascinated with health, nutrition, and herbs. I was obsessed with nature and its ability to create seemingly perfect medicinals. Plants weren't just pretty to look at, plants helped heal the human body! This realization prompted me to enroll in a master's program in acupuncture and herbalism. I studied traditional Chinese medicine for four years, learning about

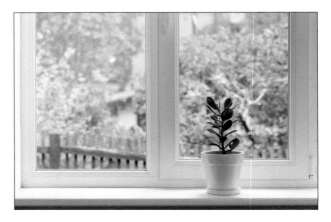

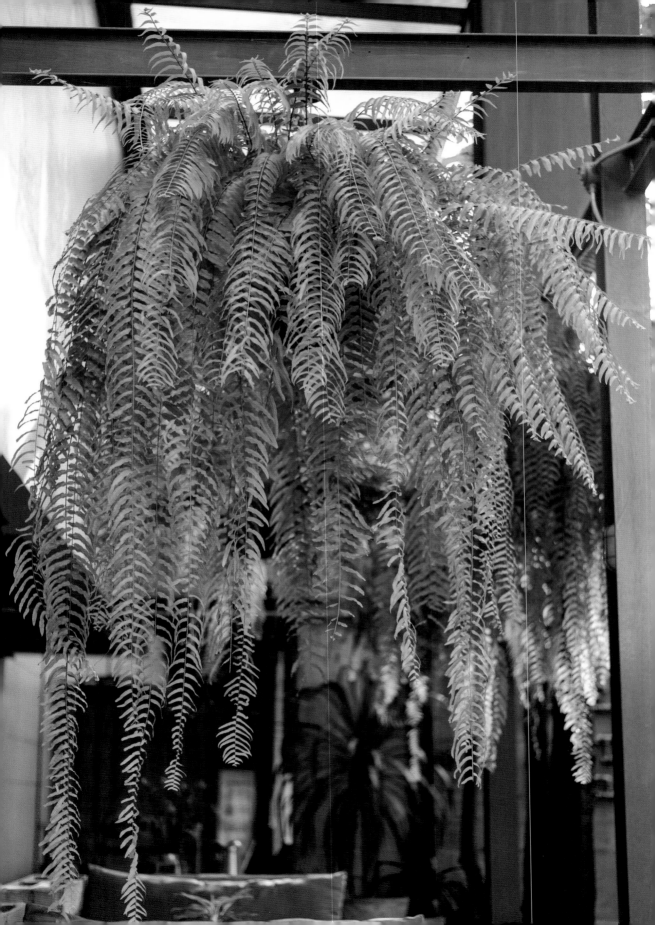

more than four hundred types of plants and hundreds of herbal formulas—and how to identify, categorize, utilize, and heal with herbs.

It was my herbal education that really propelled me out of my plant-killing rut. I decided that if I wanted to be a true herbalist, one who utilized the plants I grew for medicinal purposes, I needed to learn how to grow them and keep them alive. It seemed like an unattainable task: How many times could I fail before I succeeded? The answer? A ton.

I read every book on gardening I could get my hands on, devoured every blog post, asked every person who kept a plant alive for more than three months for advice, and got back into the gardening game. I went to the nurseries and plant stores, bought myself the easiest plants to grow, and the learning began. For the first time ever I was keeping my plants alive, and, dare I say, they were thriving! I think I could say I got my gardening groove back, but to be honest I never had a gardening groove to begin with.

My herbal knowledge had somehow ignited my innate gardening abilities. They were hidden deep inside my failed gardener exterior, and I was becoming skilled. I started accumulating more plants, and utilizing them for medicinal purposes. My aloe plant wasn't just a fixture on my windowsill, it was my ointment for scrapes, bruises, and sunburns. My chamomile wasn't just a pretty display of white flowers and sweet-smelling aromas, it was my cure for restless sleep and anxiety. The purple lavender sitting on my kitchen table wasn't just an added sprig of color, it was my stress relief medicinal.

I started creating my own homemade remedies and medicinals. First, it simply meant making tea out of my fresh herbal leaves, proudly sipping my boring mint tea with a grin of accomplishment on my face. Slowly I began to experiment, adding in oils, spices, and other odd ingredients to create salves for my skin, lip balm, or tinctures.

The plants in my home became more to me than just decor; they became a part of my health routine. Houseplants are amazing fixtures to any home, office, or room. They bring forth radiant displays of color, joy, and health benefits. And if you aren't interested in cultivating plants for medicinal purposes, it doesn't matter. They still provide us with a wide array of benefits to our health, mentally and physically. They actually might be the ultimate health supplement for the millions of us who forget to take our actual vitamins and refuse to eat kale.

It may have taken me years to cultivate my skills for growing and nurturing plants, but my love and passion for these flowering displays of nature kept me going. House-plants are a sure way to nurture your health, decorate your home, and make you feel better without really trying. So when it comes to creating your own indoor garden, don't let a few broken plants keep you down; you'll grow your green thumb eventually.

—Michelle Polk, LAc

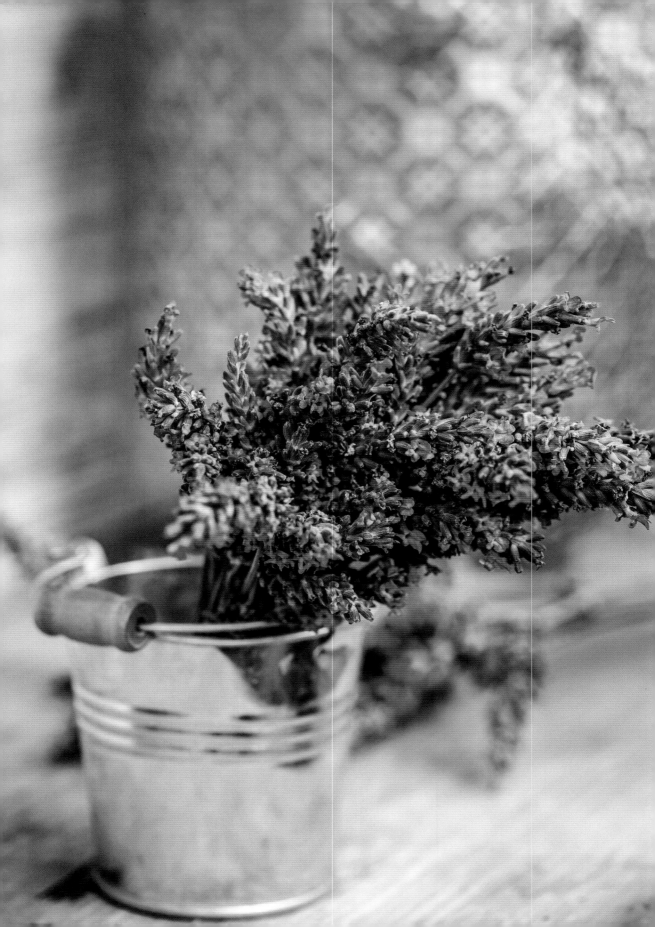

PART I

Why You Should Care About Plants and Herbs

"If you've never experienced the joy of accomplishing
more than you can, plant a garden."
—Robert Brault

"I thought I was cool until I realized plants can eat sun and poop out air."
—Jim Bugg

"Look deep into nature and then you will understand everything better."
—Albert Einstein

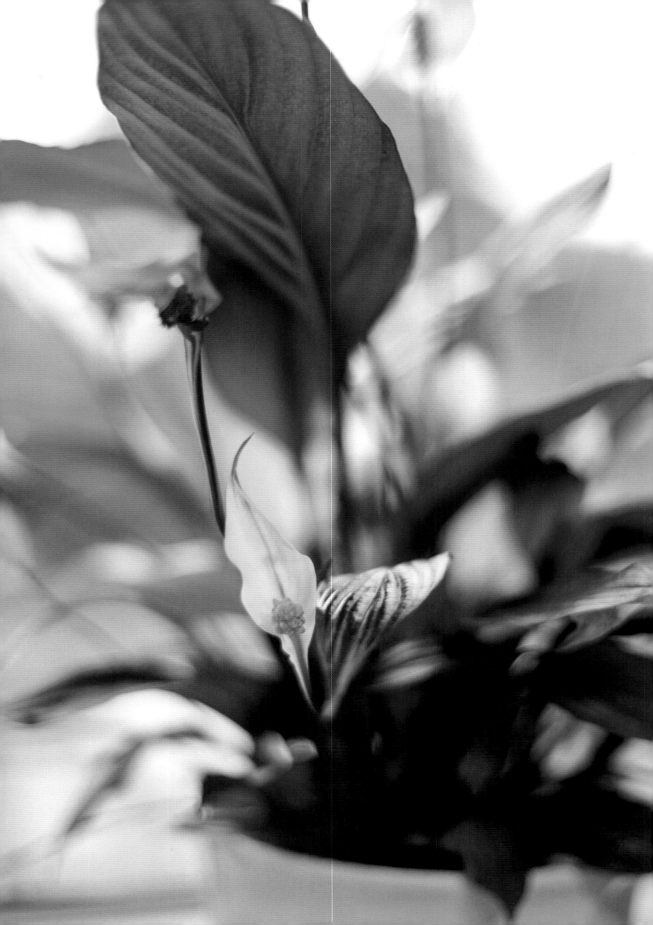

Chapter One: Houseplants for Your Health

Houseplants may conjure up thoughts of pleasant decor, added elements of design recommended by your favorite HGTV show, or background noise to an already busy home. The green and colorful flora aren't often thought of as much more than permanent fixtures on your grandmother's kitchen table, or some added kitsch to your neighbor's living room. But how often do you think of your jade plant as a health supplement? When was the last time you thanked your English ivy fern for filtering your air or reducing your stress? Or when did you last look at your philodendron and thank it for helping you concentrate and focus for an exam?

Plants are some of the healthiest additions you could add to your home, and you don't even have to ingest them. The simple act of having plants can help you heal more quickly, sleep better, focus more intently, reduce stress levels, boost the immune system, reduce depression levels, and more. And it's possible to reap these immense health benefits just by having these seemingly innocuous displays of nature sit in your house, doing absolutely nothing but look pretty.

Forget the dreaded agony of waking up at five in the morning to run three miles or the horror of meal planning based on a point system. Health is more than just following strict guidelines that are rare to achieve. Health is the accumulation of all your lifestyle choices, which include the addition of plants to your home.

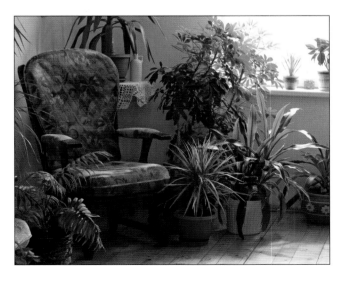

With the advent of technology—computers, iPhones, smart homes, smart watches, smart cars, or really anything that begins with the word *smart*—we've drifted further away from the natural world in which we evolved. The "nature" we've become accustomed to involves trees purposely planted along sidewalks or lawns, perfectly manicured in quaint neighborhoods. Most of us live in cities with little reminders of the natural world, often going days or weeks without stepping on grass or acknowledging a tree. The concrete jungles in which we live are a far cry from the forests and natural habitats of our ancestors. And the times we purposely set foot in nature (camping, for example) we still choose to stay inside, protected from the great outdoors. Car camping has become the ultimate retreat into nature, or into our hatchbacks.

We too often forget that humans evolved in nature alongside plants, and we depended on the flora and fauna for survival. Humans needed plants for their nutrition, healing properties, oxygen, and other features for clothes, shelter, resins, oils, food, and even customs and religious rites. Plants, on the other hand, are way more independent than we are—they appreciate our carbon dioxide output and possibly our ability to spread their seed, but they'd happily survive without us. As technology continually speeds up, catapulting us into space, creating for us newer and more exciting cars, homes, video games, and virtual reality, it will be humans who end up on the losing side of this reality. This alienation from the natural world is making us more depressed, stressed, chronically ill, and unhappy. And it's only getting worse. With the effects of climate change increasing, we are seeing a decimation of the natural world, our forests and oceans, rivers and valleys, and a loss of the many plants we have so depended on for our survival.

But don't get too depressed yet. While some issues seem so extravagantly large we can feel paralyzed, the most important thing to do is start right at home. Get one of your favorite plants out, place it next to you, and read on to understand why your beautiful ponytail fern makes you so happy. Because the only solution to mankind living inside is to bring the plants with us.

Improved Air Quality

Do you want to look younger, sleep better, reduce your stress, lower your depression, heal faster, and improve your focus? If you answered yes, there's good news. You can get all these amazing benefits without going to the doctor! In fact, plants are so good for you, if you could bottle up all their amazing benefits into a pill, it would be a billion-dollar blockbuster. The first major benefit you receive from plants is better air. Yes, plants are able to filter contaminants and toxins out of our air, making us healthier and preventing costly long-term illnesses from appearing in the first place.

Humans spend a whopping 90 percent of their lives indoors, mostly in their homes, continually breathing in recycled air. Our cultural allergy to the outdoors is providing us with a unique experience of a myriad of physical reactions to our

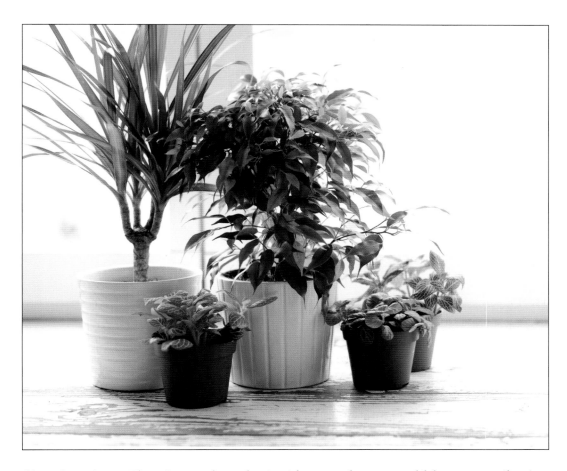

dirty interiors. The air you breathe inside your home could be a contributing factor to a variety of illnesses, and more damaging than the air in the most polluted cities. From frequent colds to dry skin, chronic cough, eye irritation, and memory lapse, the stagnant particles we call "air" are making us sick. There's even a term for this phenomenon called "sick building syndrome." Very original.

Virtually every home is overrun with a variety of toxic pollutants, including carbon monoxide, hydrocarbons, chemicals in pesticides, paints, cleaners, deodorants, hairsprays, laundry detergents, fireplaces, rugs, clothing, sheets, off-gases from furniture, carpets, glue, and even your air fresheners. **Newsflash: Your ocean breeze–scented air fresheners are in fact synthetic, toxic pollutants, and their smell resembles the interior of your last Uber ride rather than the actual ocean.**

Air quality is pertinent to good health, and if we are continually breathing in pollutants, we're putting ourselves at risk for serious long-term health complications such as asthma, cancer, and other chronic illnesses. While not often talked about, this public health issue is something which needs to be addressed. Luckily, going to your nearest garden center is an easy way to prevent the harms of our indoor lifestyle. A good rule of thumb is to have a clean-air plant for every one hundred square feet of your home.

The NASA Clean Air Study

Even NASA understood the importance of our leafy friends, conducting a study[1] in 1989 examining their ability to clean and filter the air for space stations, and what they found was impressive. The research demonstrated that common houseplants not only recycle our air, absorbing the carbon dioxide we breathe out while releasing precious oxygen back into our atmosphere, but they also have the ability to filter out carcinogenic chemicals, such as benzene, formaldehyde, trichloroethylene, ammonia, and xylene. But how?

Plants absorb carbon dioxide and also particulates in the air, which are then processed into the life-affirming oxygen we breathe in, but that's not the whole story. There are also microorganisms in the potting soil that are responsible for a big part of this cleaning effect. You heard it, the dirt that we so often avoid touching is the very dirt that is keeping us healthy and saving our lungs from toxic compounds. The leaves, roots, soil, and all the microorganisms of a plant have a part to play in their ability to clean our precious air, and every plant we place inside our airtight homes is another win for our air quality.

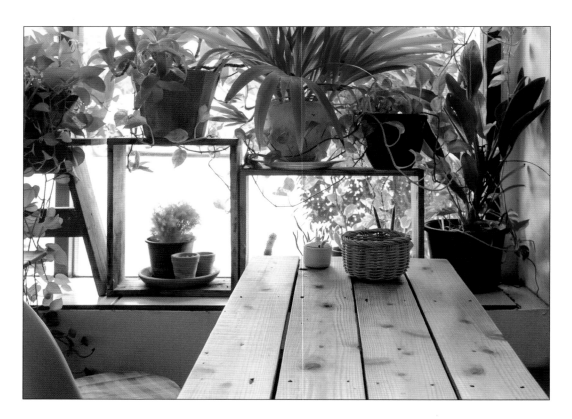

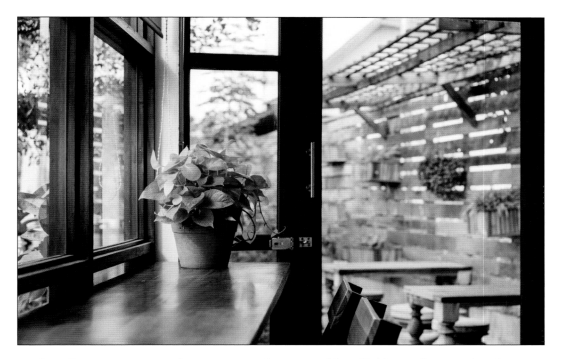

One Japanese researcher went as far as to identify how these microbes are affecting our health, and what he found will change the way you look at tree huggers. Forests are more than just trees and dirt; they are an ecosystem filled with airborne antifungal and antibacterial compounds called phytoncides.[2] It seems as though when you inhale these compounds, they boost your white blood cells, especially a type which attacks tumors and viruses. Taking a hike reduces cancer, and not in the way you'd imagine. Forget cardio, bring me more phytoncides! For those of us who don't have regular access to a forest for a daily hike, we can still get the benefits of microbes from our indoor gardens. High five!

So while we're trying to inhale certain microbes and bacteria, what should we be avoiding and what are the top chemicals that our homegrown friends are able to filter away? The following is a list of the most common indoor air pollutants, ones that are easily filtered away by clean-air plants.

The Most Common Indoor Air Pollutants

Benzene: A widely known carcinogen often found in gasoline fumes, cigarettes, and car exhausts, and used in industries related to plastic, oil, gasoline, rubber, and more. What's startling is that benzene is found at high levels in indoor air, which could be from car exhaust, paints, adhesives, and even in your new furniture. The more time you spend indoors could equal the more exposure you have to benzene. The World Health Organization states that exposure to benzene is a major public health concern, citing exposure can lead to cancer and aplastic anemia.

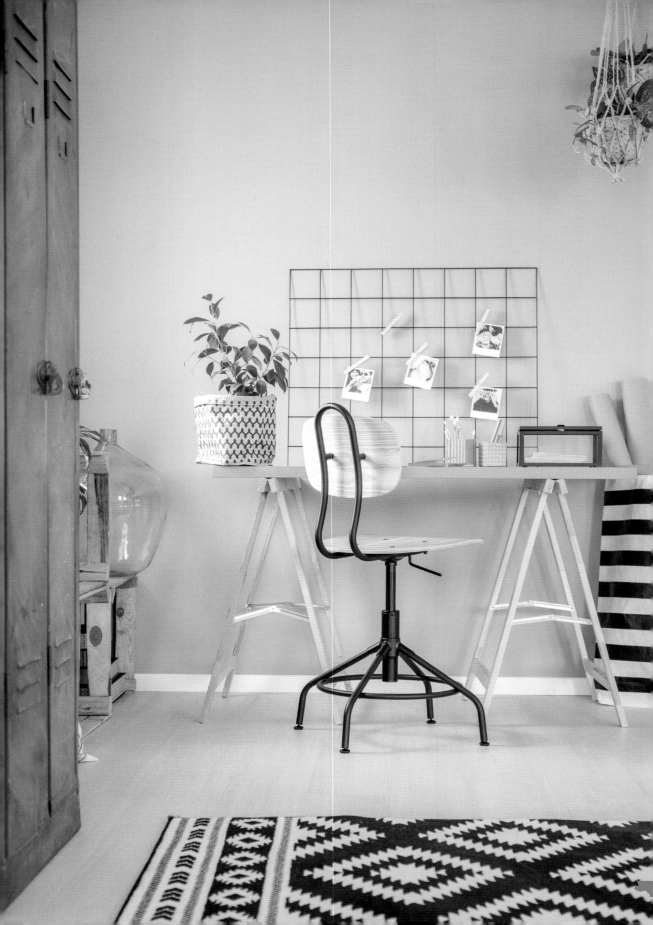

Formaldehyde: Another widely known chemical, this colorless, flammable, strong-smelling gas is found in a variety of household products and building materials. Often used in glues; adhesives; wood products such as particleboard, plywood, and fiberboard; and fungicides, germicides, and disinfectants. The Environmental Protection Agency states that formaldehyde can cause short-term irritations of the skin, eyes, nose, and throat, and high levels of exposure may cause some types of cancers.

Trichloroethylene: Another chemical commonly used as an industrial solvent. Chronic exposure has been linked to cancer and other chronic illnesses.

Ammonia: One of the most widely produced chemicals in the United States, ammonia is actually found in nature and is produced in the human body. Often found in fertilizer and the manufacturing of plastics, explosives, fabrics, pesticides, dyes, and other chemicals, you're most likely exposed to it via your household cleaning solutions. Overexposure to this chemical can cause irritation; burns; eye, nose, and throat irritation; and lung damage.

Xylene: Widely used as a chemical solvent, cleaning agent, and paint thinner, xylene has been shown to cause irritation to the mouth and throat, dizziness, headache, confusion, and liver and kidney damage.

Plants may appear docile, but their ability to filter out harmful substances and chemicals from your air proves that their strength is more than meets the eye. According to NASA, some houseplants are better than others at cleaning and filtering our air; below are the ten best plants to add to your polluted home (I'm not judging).

My Top Ten Favorite Plants to Filter the Air

Boston Fern

If you're looking for a dependable presence in your life, search no further. The Boston fern is the ultimate houseplant, a favorite of indoor gardeners since the Victorian age. The good old fern ranks number nine in NASA's top fifty air purifying plants list, and is the most efficient at removing formaldehyde from the air, not to mention its ability to remove other contaminants.

English Ivy

English ivy is a workhorse when it comes to cleaning your air, filtering out trichloroethylene, formaldehyde, benzene, and xylene. It also amazingly clears out fecal matter from the air, so you're in luck if you have any pets or children! This vine looks beautiful in a hanging pot or around your windowsill, and will make you look way more elegant. This is a great plant for beginners and is easy to take care of. However, be careful if you have pets, as it can cause problems for both dogs and cats.

Golden Pothos

Also known as Devil's ivy, the golden pothos is one of my favorite houseplants due to its indestructible nature. This plant thrives on neglect, and if you are new to indoor gardening, start with the classic pothos. The golden pothos also does an amazing job of filtering the air of formaldehyde, xylene, toluene, benzene, carbon monoxide, and more.

Peace Lily

The name alone should make you want to grab one of these plants for your home. What's better is that NASA found the peace lily to be one of the top three plants for removing indoor air toxins, such as ammonia, formaldehyde, and benzene. However, the peace lily is toxic to animals and children. Keep it away from reach, as it can cause skin irritation, burning, and swelling.

Spider Plant

The ever interesting spider plant will eliminate formaldehyde and xylene from your air and grows very quickly indoors. If you're lucky, it'll even produce beautiful white blossoms. This plant is nontoxic.

Snake Plant

Despite its name, I truly love the snake plant for its ease of care and very unique look. A classic houseplant often used in offices for its ability to survive in low light or artificial light environments, the snake plant has been found to clean out benzene, formaldehyde, trichloroethylene, and xylene.

Chinese Evergreen

The Chinese evergreen is one of the most beautiful and unique-looking houseplants around. Native to tropical forests in Asia, these plants can filter out benzene, carbon monoxide, formaldehyde, trichloroethylene, and more! However, this is toxic to dogs, so make sure to keep it out of their reach.

Flamingo Lily

One of the more unique and beautiful houseplants, the flamingo lily is easy to grow and will thrive for many years on your kitchen table if provided with ideal conditions. It should be kept away from pets, children, or any adult who acts like a child, as it contains calcium oxalate crystals, which can be harmful if chewed. Flamingo lilies been found to filter formaldehyde, ammonia, and xylene.

Aloe Vera

Not just for your skin anymore! Aloe vera has been found to filter out formaldehyde from the air. Aloe is also very easy to maintain, only requiring watering when the soil is dry. The leaves hold a fluid which is known to be an anti-inflammatory and to possess wound healing properties!

Bamboo Palm

An overachiever when it comes to filtering formaldehyde out of the air, the bamboo palm can grow to be as tall as twelve feet high, making it one of the most efficient air filters around. The bamboo palm also removes benzene, as well as trichloroethylene, and is a pet-friendly plant.

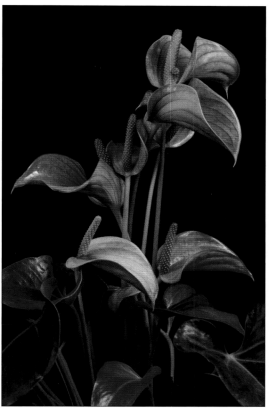

A flamingo lily in full bloom.

With so many options, our air doesn't have to make us sick anymore. It's clear now that we can't live in the vacuum of our tidy, chemical-laden homes. It's not possible to thrive indoors without plants, and in order to live healthy lives, we must bring nature with us. Luckily for us, many plants can thrive indoors with us, helping us breathe cleaner air and making our homes beautiful representations of health and wellness.

Plants Lower Stress and Depression

Stress is all too common in our contemporary lifestyles. From traffic jams, long and boring commutes, the twenty-four-hour news cycle, and the constant pings of emails and cell phones to the never ending break of social media and the Internet, it's no wonder we're all about to burst a communal blood vessel. Life may be getting more efficient, but it sure isn't getting any easier, or happier. Don't get me wrong, we are living in very exciting times, but *Dancing with the Stars* is not a cure for depression, it's just a distraction from our hectic lives.

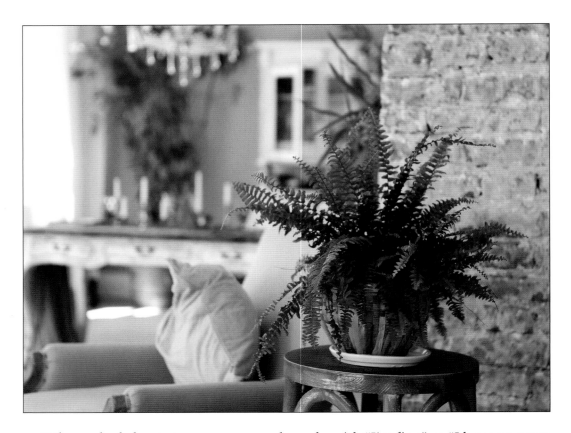

When asked about stress many people reply with "I'm fine" or "I have no more stress than anyone else!" This is not a good sign. Our criterion of stress should not be how you compare to your next-door neighbor, Joe, who works seventy hours a week and drinks five gin and tonics to unwind. In fact, forget everyone you know because chances are they're all stress balls who don't know the definition of relaxation.

Let's get dramatic for a second: stress is killing you. It's one of the main causes of 60 percent of all human illnesses and disease, such as heart attack, stroke, and heart disease. How is this so? Well, the body can't distinguish between the stress of getting cut off by another BMW on your way to work, or the stress of being chased by a mountain lion. This means your body reacts just as strongly to a seeming annoyance as an actual life-threatening situation.

The problem with this scenario is that these stressful occurrences are happening on a daily basis, constantly pinging your nervous system and flooding your body with hormones meant to be used only in times of actual, dire need. Long-term and chronic exposure to stress disrupts nearly every system of your body, suppressing the immune system, increasing heart rate and blood pressure, contributing to infertility and irritable bowel syndrome (IBS), and even rewiring your brain to be more prone to anxiety and depression.

And stress isn't the only cause of depression. There are many variables that contribute to depression, including genetics, life circumstances, grief, changes in hormone levels, and newer research pointing towards the gut biome and nutrition. According to the National Institute of Mental Health, 16 million adults had at least one major depressive episode in 2012, or around 6.9 percent of the population. And that's reported cases. According to the World Health Organization, more than 350 million people suffer from depression worldwide.

Depression is a huge topic, with many causes and many types; however, it's generally known to suck. This is some stressful news, but there are some remedies to help. With that said, plants have been shown to increase levels of happiness, lower levels of stress, and lower the incidence of depression. The unseen mental benefits of plants is yet another reason to add some greenery to your home and start gardening.

Research from the Norwegian University of Life Sciences and Uppsala University in Sweden found that the mere presence of plants in an office or home increased levels of happiness, reduced stress and fatigue, and reduced the amount of sick leave workers took.[3] An-

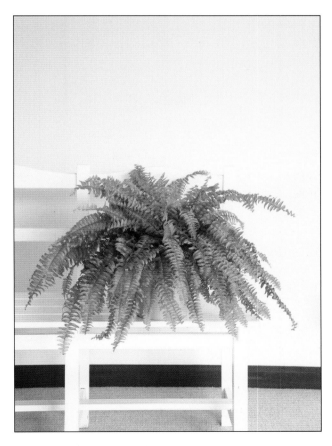

other study found that indoor plants may reduce psychological stress by suppressing the sympathetic nervous system (our fight-or-flight response), making us less stressed and our bodies more relaxed.[4]

Even more research found that when plants are placed in already high-stress work environments, people reported feeling calmer and experienced an increased sense of happiness. Having contact with nature, whether it be indoor plants, increased visibility of nature, or even better access to parks or outdoor spaces, improved health promotion efforts and reduced perceived stress, and general health complaints decreased. Just thirty minutes of walking surrounded by the natural world reduced depression in 71 percent of partici-pants![5]

In fact, the research keeps pointing back to nature leading to happiness in humans. A 2010 study[6] found that hiking or walking through the forest for two hours per day over a two-day period lowered stress hormone levels, blood pressure, and pulse rate. And science is showing that just being able to see a natural setting with your own two eyes increases your brain's pleasure receptors. Add a hot tub and some bubbly, and you'll be the happiest you've ever been in your life.

Plants Increase Focus

While technology is increasing at lightning speeds, our focus is dwindling at the speed of sound. Yes, we carry minicomputers in our back pockets, travel the world via virtual reality, and drive high-performance electric vehicles. However, it seems as though we can't get through a conversation anymore without checking our Instagram, our ability to read a book dwindles in comparison to our Netflix bingeing abilities, and our listening skills only last for approximately 2.1 seconds.

According to a new study from Microsoft[7], humans now lose focus after eight seconds, one second less than our goldfish competition. Our increased depen-

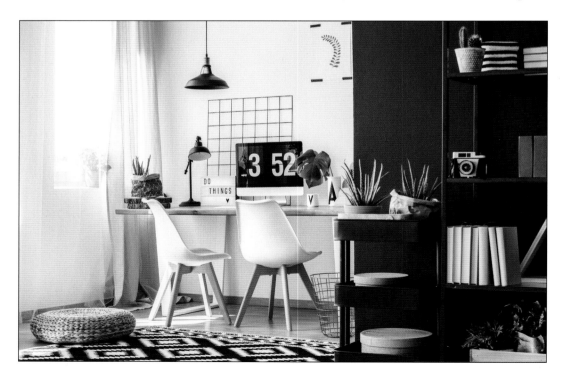

dence on Google, GPS systems, and everything in between has made us less focused, impatient, and perhaps a little dumber. Since the year 2000, our attention spans have dropped from an average of twelve seconds down to eight, and our minds are constantly waiting for the next *bing, click, ping, beep* from our phones, emails, and computers. Good luck getting through this book; if you make it to the end, make sure to congratulate yourself!

There's good news, however, for those of us who love plants. We're beginning to understand that the mere presence of plants in our workplace or home environment can drastically change how we think and how we focus. One study published in the *Journal of Environmental Psychology* found that having plants in your workspace can boost your ability to focus and maintain attention.[8] The human mind can stare at boring spreadsheets and Google docs for only so long, and don't get started on expense reports and billing—we can only do so much. Our brains are complicated biocomputers, and we have only a limited capacity for what is known as "directed attention." Directed attention basically means anything we do at work: controlled, focused, concentrated attention. And of course, it diminishes the more we use it in a day. No wonder Google has ping-pong tables and nap pods at its workplace!

With this in mind, when we engage with nature, walk in a park, or look at plants in our office, our mind is able to continually draw its attention to something new—a leaf, a blade of grass, a bird pooping on a stranger. Your senses are continually being engaged, capturing your attention over and over again. This second kind of attention is known as "undirected attention." Undirected attention allows us to rest our directed minds and rejuvenate for the next round of intense, directed thinking. Plants are some of the most effective ways to bring forward our undirected minds, thus leading us to a more focused work day.

Other studies[9] have looked specifically at plants in the workplace, comparing sparse desks with those decorated with your average fern or snake plant. What they found was that people who sat at a desk with flowers and plants were better at paying attention to a task than those sitting at an empty, lonely desk. The restorative breaks that plants give us should not be underestimated. Imagine a world where every classroom was a mini jungle and every office resembled a beautiful forest. These oases would provide us with the ability to work more diligently, learn more intently, and happily focus on our next task.

Plants Speed Up Healing

When it comes to recovering from an injury there are plenty of things we can do to speed up the process: physical therapy, sleep, baths, sunlight, vitamins, Netflix binges, and eating your broccoli are just a few. And while you may be aware of the many health benefits of ingesting plants and herbs, you might not realize the vast benefits of just placing one next to your bed while healing from an injury. Don't worry, I'm not making you eat your Boston fern.

In fact, it's been shown that adding plants to a health care environment not only makes patients less stressed and anxious but also improves healing times. Just three to five minutes spent looking at nature (trees, flowers, grass, birds) began to reduce anger, pain, muscle tension, and heart and brain electrical activity.

One study found that viewing plants during the recovery period had a positive influence and was directly linked to health outcomes of surgical patients. The findings confirmed that patients who had flowers and plants in their recovery rooms had lower blood pressure, lower levels of pain (and thus reduced medication), and reduced anxiety and fatigue compared to patients who had no plants at all. Additionally, the majority of patients who had plants in their rooms noted that the most positive quality of their recovery rooms were the plants themselves. The patients who didn't have plants in their rooms mentioned the television as being the most favorable part of their rooms.[10] Nature wins out every time.

But the most exciting part of this is how plants can be present and useful for the whole healing process, aiding in every step of recovery. The study found that as patients started feeling better, they began to engage more with their plants, such as watering, pruning, and general upkeep. This allowed them to get out of bed and interact with something unrelated to the hospital, and unrelated to recovery. The best part is this only decreased healing times, as the patients were moving and progressing faster than those who had no plants to care for.[11]

Nature is making a comeback in the health world, with many more hospitals opting to have specially designed outdoor spaces for hospital patients and assisted-living residents. While hospitals may bring forth imagery of a sterile, uninviting environment, or that place you went to when you accidentally cut your finger open with a box cutter, things are starting to change. Humans know innately the positive effects of sunlight, walking through a forest or garden, putting our hands in the dirt, or hearing birds chirping outside our window. But now, science is starting to prove it.

It wasn't until 1984 when researchers started looking into the beneficial effects of gardens and plants on the healing process, and in that research they were able to demonstrate that viewing a garden can speed healing from surgery, infections, and other illnesses. And you don't necessarily have to have plants in your room to benefit—just having a window which looks out onto a garden or trees has increased benefits than those who merely looked out onto a brick wall or a parking lot.

What's great about this interest in nature and healing is that hospitals are beginning to listen and understand that they are some of the biggest sources of stress. These loud, smelly, sterile, scary centers of "healing" more accurately are centers of fright rather than serene healing oases. Who's ever walked into a hospital and said, "Gosh, I'm so glad I'm here!" When stressed, our immune systems decrease, pain levels increase, and healing times take longer. How can we heal in rooms that remind us of illness, wasting, awful odors, and fast-paced melancholy? And patients aren't the only ones who benefit from these displays of nature—hospital employees are sometimes the people who need this restful distraction the most.

It's no question that nature helps us heal. We feel more grounded, relaxed, and present when we are engaging with plants, flowers, trees, and the like. Houseplants are amazing ways to bring nature indoors, allowing us to placate our need to be surrounded by the very thing we are distancing ourselves from—the outdoors. Humans need nature, and even if you live in the concrete jungle, there are many ways in which you can participate with our natural friends. And it's super easy too!

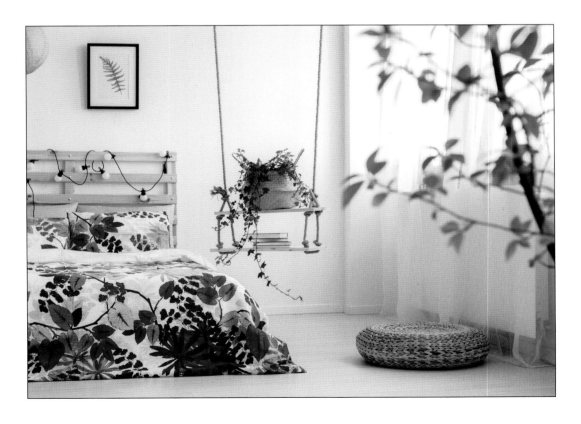

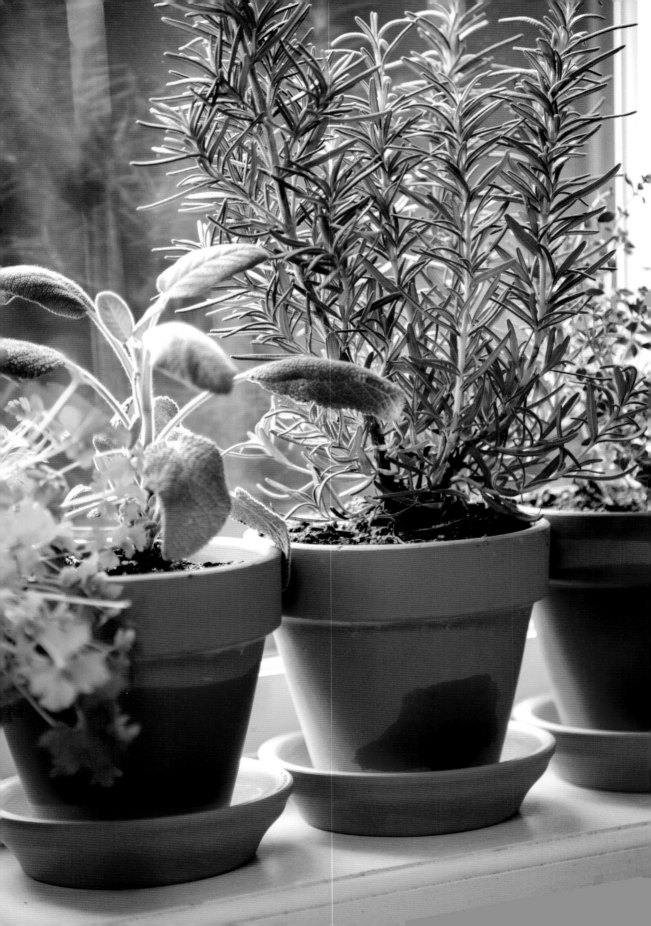

Chapter Two: Why Everyone Should Be Taking Herbs. Yes, Even You.

It may come as no surprise that I love plants. They are beautiful, mysterious, glamorous, and miraculous living things that not only look good but heal! These tiny healers can make someone feel better within moments of being in their presence. But let's get real—the majority of a plant's ability to heal comes from ingesting them or using them directly on the body. They can only do so much standing in the corner of your living room for your midcentury modern condo decor.

Herbal medicine has been increasing in popularity over the past several years with more and more people understanding the importance of taking control of their health and using natural methods for preventative care. That being said,

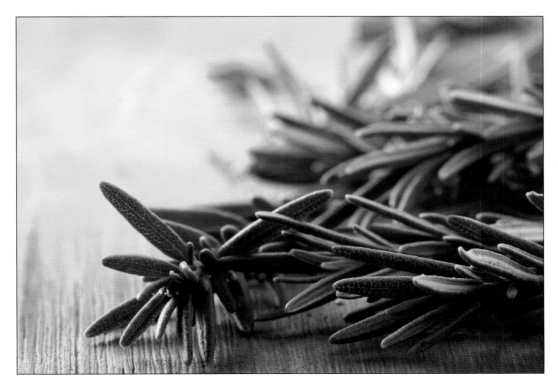

herbal medicine has been around for over five thousand years, with every culture showcasing some sort of herbal/folk medicinal knowledge—this isn't just some hipster fad. Herbs have been shown to have incredible effects on the body, including anti-inflammatory, antibacterial, antiviral, antifungal, cancer preventing, pain reducing, gut enhancing, and other healing properties. When part of a daily routine, herbs can provide amazing benefits to your mind and body.

As an herbalist, I get very excited about herbs. Yes, they are tasty in your favorite slow cooker recipe, and they are beautiful garnishes to your coq au vin. But as an herbalist I'm trained to look deeper into your basil plant, rosemary sprig, and even the dandelion growing incessantly over your nearest soccer field. And before you spray your so-called weeds with Monsanto's next poisonous products, why not take a little time to understand how amazing your mint truly is. Hint: mint isn't just for mojitos anymore!

A Very Brief History of Herbal Medicine

Herbal medicine has been around since before recorded history, with Chinese, Babylonian, Native American, Indian, and Egyptian cultures swigging down gross herbal, dirt-tasting concoctions as early as 3000 BC. And it was the monks during the medieval ages who carried the tradition of herbalism, growing medicinal herbs and serving as the medical schools of their time.

Chinese herbalism is the third-oldest form of medicine, only following the Egyptian and Babylonian medical traditions. The discovery of the oldest known list of medicinal herbs can be attributed to the legendary emperor Shen Nung in what is called the *Shennong Ben Cao Jing* (ca. 3000 BC). Named the father of Chinese agriculture and leader of the ancient clan, he literally tasted hundreds, if not thousands, of herbs to test the medicinal properties of each plant and to determine which were safe and which were poisonous. Talk about being a team player . . . there's no *I* in *herb*.

This rich tradition of herbalism was created from the detailed observation of nature with trial and error, together leading to thousands of years of case studies and proven remedies.

Be it Western or Eastern herbalism, the ancient Chinese, Indians, Egyptians, Babylonians, or Native Americans, all traditions were passed down from generation to generation, healer to apprentice, professor to student.

There are hundreds of thousands of species of plants known today, with more being discovered every year. Countless unknown plants exist in the world unbeknownst to us, and with healing properties yet to be discovered. Some herbalists go as far as to believe for every human illness that exists, so too does a plant which is able to cure it.

And while hundreds of years ago humans regularly ingested more than one hundred species of herbs to keep them healthy, today it's down to ten to twenty. We are missing out on the integral elements of nutrition and health-promoting parts of our diet and lifestyle. No wonder there's an epidemic of chronic illness—our bodies don't have the necessary tools to work properly. How many of us make sure our cars get the right fuel, oil, and care in order to make sure they run smoothly for as long as possible. For many of us, we expect our bodies to run without a hitch, but without the same maintenance, care, and proper fuel.

Thanks Aspirin . . . Er, Willow Bark!

Herbs come in all shapes, sizes, pronunciations, aromas, and more likely than not, gross taste. You've probably heard of mint, lavender, rosemary, and even dandelions, but have you ever heard of rhodiola, turkey tail, reishi, or chaste tree? What about feverfew, schisandra, wormwood, or mugwort? All of these unique, fake-sounding names may remind you of Harry Potter but are actually real, immensely healing, powerful herbal plants that can be used for a variety of aches, pains, illnesses, and more. In fact, many of your favorite over-the-counter remedies originally came from plants and herbs; I'm talking about you, aspirin!

The pharmaceutical industry can thank nature for many of their newest blockbuster drugs or miracle remedies. In the past twenty-five years, around 70 percent of new drugs came from Mother Nature. Despite all our attempts for

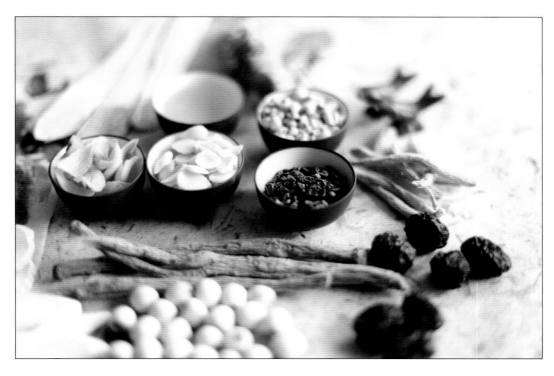

synthetic medicines and our need to create superior products, Mother Nature always has the most sophisticated answers for our health ills.

One of humankind's favorite over-the-counter medicines exists because of the willow tree. You've probably popped a few for your hangover, headache, or daily regimen to prevent a heart attack, not even realizing that a pill which makes your hangover tolerable wouldn't be around if someone a long time ago hadn't decided to eat bark. Recent research has shown that aspirin can not only prevent heart attacks and strokes, but a twenty-year study found that it also reduced the risk of cancer by at least 20 percent.[12] No, this didn't just all of a sudden appear from some lab created by a mad scientist in a white coat; it actually has been used for thousands of years by various cultures, but in its whole-plant form.

The use of aspirin's active ingredient dates back to the ancient Egyptians, who used the plant for aches and pains, and the great Greek physician Hippocrates stated that willow bark helped relieve fevers and pain. But it wasn't until the 1800s that researchers were able to identify the active ingredient in willow bark, salicylic acid. It was a chemist in the 1890s who used the form of aspirin we know today. Felix Hoffman worked for Bayer in Germany and used aspirin to help with his father's rheumatism. It was in 1899 that Bayer started distributing a powder with acetylsalicylic acid to doctors to give to their patients. It wasn't long after that it started becoming available over the counter.

But aspirin isn't the only drug that can thank a plant for its existence. For example, Taxol, one of the strongest cancer drugs on the market, was derived from the bark of the Pacific yew tree, and the groundbreaking antibiotic penicillin was derived from penicillium mold. Then there's the periwinkle plant from Madagascar, which increased the rate of remission for childhood leukemia up to 95 percent by 1997 compared to the 10 percent remission rate in 1960. This plant alone has saved over 100,000 lives. There's also the malaria drug artemisinin, made from the artemisia plant, which won Chinese scientist Youyou Tu the 2015 Nobel Prize in Physiology or Medicine.

Youyou Tu discovered artemisia as a means to help cure malaria by reading ancient Chinese medical texts. Before her discovery, over 240,000 compounds around the world had been tested, but nothing seemed to work. It wasn't until she read the old text originating from around 400 AD, where she discovered sweet wormwood was an option to treat the disease. Her team tested extracts of the herb to no effect, that is until she followed the original ancient text's exact recipe—heating the extract without allowing it to reach boiling point. Her diligence and forethought saved millions of lives. And by taking ancient wisdom to the future, she was able to harness what humans already knew thousands of years ago and convert it into modern medicine.

How Nature Provided Us with Antibiotics and How It Will Save Us from Antibiotics

The newest terrifying topic on everyone's minds is antibiotic resistance. Doomsday seems closer and closer as more and more researchers are proclaiming we are almost to the dead zone when it comes to antibiotic use. Zombies aren't going to kill us, simple infections will.

Imagine cutting yourself while attempting to break open an unusually stubborn package of Hot Pockets with your sharpest knife, only to find that your cut needs stitches. You go to the hospital and are terrified that you have an infection—not because of the costs, but because antibiotics no longer work. Any infection could equal death. Yes, this might sound dramatic, but this is the path we are headed towards, and no one wants to die from Hot Pockets.

Since the discovery of penicillin in 1928 from the penicillium mold, we've thrived and basked in the glorious wonders of antibiotics. For nearly one hundred years we haven't had to worry about infections such as rheumatic fever, pneumonia, or gonorrhea. But, oops, in 2016 the World Health Organization said that gonorrhea might soon be untreatable. And this is just one of the many infections and diseases that will become resistant to treatment. Every year, 63,000 patients in the US and 25,000 patients in the European Union die from hospital-acquired, antibiotic-resistant infections, and this number is only increasing. The global review on antimicrobial resistance stated that if we are unable to find

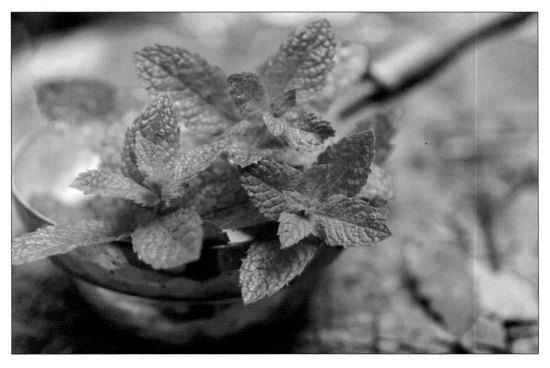

an alternative to tackle these resistant infections, ten million people will die by 2050 due to antibiotic-resistant infections.

But how did this happen? It's a simple case of overuse and denial. Oh yeah, we are great at denial. Alexander Fleming, the man who discovered penicillin, warned us of this depressing fate knowing all too well the effects of overusing this magical drug way back in the 1930s. The reason is simple. Bacteria goes through the same process of natural selection as humans. Those that survive adapt and multiply, and thus their genes are the ones passed down through generations.

Every time you take an antibiotic, not only are the microbes which caused your illness killed off, but so are the good ones which protect your body from infection. But not every single microbe is actually killed, and these bacteria are known as the resistant bacteria. Without the protection of your security team (good bacteria) the resistant bacteria are able to thrive and proliferate, transferring their drug resistance to other microbes causing more problems and damage.

Every time someone takes an antibiotic, resistant bacteria are growing in numbers and thriving. And the more a whole population of people take antibiotics, the quicker the bacteria are able to mutate—not to mention you are also increasingly killing off your good microbes which can lead to other problems such as IBS, depression, and a host of chronic illnesses. But that's for another book.

Our perpetual need to throw antibiotics at any infection or illness will create one of the biggest health crises in our time. For example, chances are that the sore throat you have is NOT strep. However, a whopping 70 percent of people who go to the doctor for a sore throat will receive antibiotics even though only 20 percent of them actually have the *Streptococcus pyogenes* bacteria. That's right, 80 percent of people who get antibiotics for their sore throat don't need antibiotics. This is one of the reasons why we are in a crisis: overuse and lack of oversight.

Strep throat is not the only reason we're experiencing antibiotic resistance; our overuse of antibacterial soaps, the need to bathe ourselves in hand sanitizers, the desire to shower several times a day, the antibiotics fed to our livestock to keep them fat and juicy, and our general distrust of dirt have allowed bacteria to mutate and proliferate, creating bigger, badder strains of bacteria and resistant illness.

Don't Panic, Plants May Save Your Life

With the imminent antibiotic crisis threatening our way of life, researchers have begun to realize that maybe our way out of this mess isn't inside a lab configuring synthetic formulations. Perhaps the way to dig ourselves out of this bacterial hole

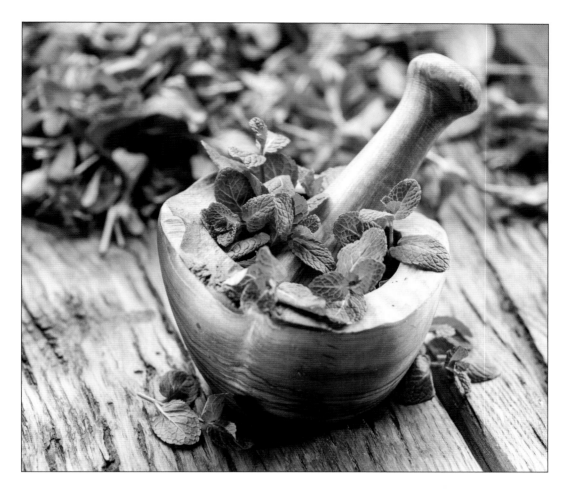

is to go the natural route. In fact, that is exactly what some researchers are doing. The future of Western medicine may in fact be ancient herbal medicine.

A number of researchers, including Dr. Cassandra Quave, an ethnobotanist from Emory University, are looking to use the knowledge of plants from ancient cultures to derive new medicines for our current needs. Traditional plant-based medicine is a treasure trove of knowledge and experience, with thousands of years of usage, trial and error, and recorded successes. However, looking to herbal medicines and ancient traditions wasn't always the fashionable choice.

Since the 1970s, the pharmaceutical industry was more interested in synthetic drug development, hoping this would be the future of medicine. It's also easier to formulate something in a lab than decipher nature's sophisticated and incredibly complex chemistry. In the words of Simon Gibbons, a medicinal phytochemist at University College London, "Nature is a super chemist. It's been doing this a lot longer than we or even mammals have been around. Plants have been doing this for around 400 million years." Talk about intimidating. Believe it or not, the immensely complex chemistry involved in keeping a plant alive has the potential to be potent medicine for humans. Because plants are literally grounded, they are unable to run or attack their predators. Instead, they create complex chemistry to poison their competition. One plant's poison is another man's potent medicine.

It's easy to forget that plants were our primary source of medicine for thousands of years. Currently, we've become so far removed from nature that you're called a hippie, woo-woo, voodoo-loving quack for trying to cure your headache with herbs. If it isn't in a pill, you must be crazy! And while a good portion of our modern medicines are derived from plants, only a small fraction of the estimated fifty thousand medicinal herbs and plants used in traditional medicines have been studied. That's a lot of wasted potential, which doesn't include the immense number of plants, herbs, and species not even discovered in the rainforests and other natural landscapes.

Recently, Dr. Cassandra Quave discovered that healers in southern Italy are using elmleaf blackberry to heal boils and abscesses. When sent to the lab, these berries were found to help prevent the staph bacteria found in abscesses from forming biofilms, which allows bacteria like methicillin-resistant *Staphlococcus aureus* to attach themselves onto medical devices and living tissue—which would allow these microbes to communicate and mutate. If we can keep the bacteria from evolving and mutating, we can make them more vulnerable and thus more treatable. This is why natural medicines are so important and unique. While humans are looking to massacre these antibiotic-resistant strains, nature is able

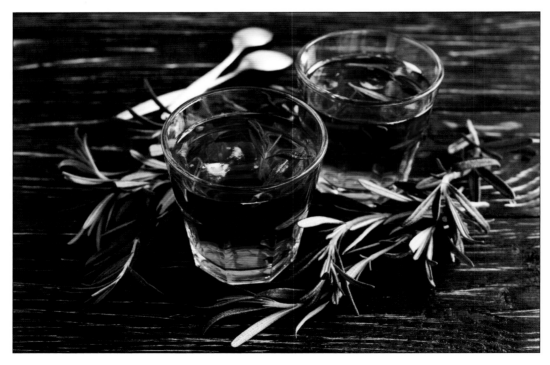

to help us look in different directions, solving the puzzle from another point of view. The berries may not have killed the staph, but they kept it from spreading, which is exactly what we need in order to stop the future resistance. The term *balance* fits in nicely here. Nature loves balance.

But there are still plenty of hurdles to overcome when it comes to using nature as a remedy. Many pharmaceuticals aren't interested in or are just plain apathetic about studying plant medicines due to their immense complexity and their less-than-stunning profit potential. If you make a pharmaceutical drug derived from a traditional herbal remedy, a percentage of the proceeds must go to the people who originally created the herbal formula, meaning that individual nations have sovereign rights over their medical traditions. So while there is incredible potential when it comes to plant medicines, the current apathy towards these potential lifesavers will have to change in order for us to reap the full benefits.

Killing the Rainforest Is Killing Our Medicine Cabinet

With all the potential medical benefits from the vast biodiversity on earth, we must also talk about how climate change and deforestation are affecting our quest for new medicines. The deforestation of tropical forests, rainforests, the Amazon, and more is contributing to the eradication of possible life-saving medicines. You can't deny yourself out of this crisis.

For example, the island of Madagascar gave us the life-saving periwinkle plant, which we talked about earlier for its ability to increase remission rates of childhood leukemia from only 10 percent in the 1960s to over 95 percent today. However, this miracle plant is under threat. Madagascar houses an incredible array of biodiversity, some 250,000 species, of which 75 percent are found nowhere else on earth! However, 90 percent of the Madagascan forests have been decimated and their rich and complex soils completely washed away. It's hard to know how many potentially life-saving, groundbreaking, medical-changing, Nobel Prize–winning remedies are completely gone.

Even worse, we have no idea what we are losing, or exactly how much we are losing. However, we can approximate the extinction rate in 2100 to be around 50 percent of all the rainforest animals, flora, and fauna. Scientists have only studied around 1 percent of the plants found in the rainforests, but over 140 of them are becoming extinct every single day. If this doesn't scare you, I'll have what you're drinking.

Latin America is losing over 4.3 million hectares of rainforest per year. Indonesia is seeing over 80 percent loss of their rainforests, with over 28 million hectares being destroyed per year. But it just doesn't stop: 70 percent of the rainforests in Laos, Cambodia, and Vietnam are being torn down, and it's estimated that Indonesia will lose all its rainforests between 2020 and 2025. Indonesia had one of the oldest and most diverse rainforests, which means we potentially lost some of the most exciting and effective medicine cabinets in the world.

And here's the kicker—we are seeing a rise in in new diseases, especially infectious, due to the increasing practice of deforestation, which could potentially be cured by the very plants we are eradicating. As we destroy forests and ecosystems, we are destroying the homes of many species of plants, animals, and insects. Being homeless, many of these insects and animals wander into civilization, carrying with them a fun assortment of infectious diseases. One discarded partially eaten fruit by an infected bat can lead to an outbreak in livestock, which can quickly jump to humans. We can thank this phenomenon for the outbreak of Ebola, AIDS, Lyme disease, West Nile, and SARS.

Sustainability is a word you've probably heard thrown around here and there, but in fact, if we want to preserve the future of medicine, we have to set forth practices of sustainability and protections. It might be profitable to cut down forests at the moment, but in the future it will only harm the common good. Luckily, interest in natural and organic products, sustainable practices, and plant medicine will only place pressure among various industries to change their practices, and for pharmaceuticals to place more stock in biodiverse medicines. As the pharmaceutical industry becomes more involved, the hope is that the economy and job opportunities will increase, which will only help to preserve such environments. If you love plants, it would be prudent to support the causes that are helping preserve our biodiversity. Who knows, your next favorite houseplant might yet be discovered.

I Want the Whole Plant and Nothing but the Plant

While focusing on the pharmaceutical potential in researching plants and herbs, we haven't talked much about the intrinsic value in the whole plants themselves. We live in a reductionist culture, taking out the parts of we think matter, studying one isolated constituent at a time, and supercharging it to an unheard of percent, which is then made into a pharmaceutical. And while we have some amazing drugs out of this system, there are still problems associated with it.

This practice can be a dangerous one, picking out which parts we deem most important and useful while discarding the rest. We're forgetting that most things in nature work synergistically, as a whole, together. It's time to talk about how the whole is greater than the sum of its parts.

When looking at the chemical constituents of a plant, many chemists or researchers will isolate out the "active ingredient" and turn it into a drug. However, the consequences of this practice can be detrimental and overlooked. Many times

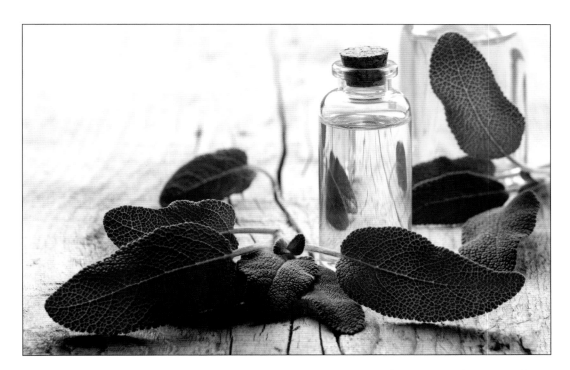

we think there is just one active ingredient working alone to make something better; however, nature doesn't work this way. Often, the whole plant and all its components work together in order to achieve a goal. This holistic approach sees the sum of the whole rather than the single, isolated approach.

Plants evolved and naturally contain substances that work together. Their phytochemistry is sophisticated, and nothing in the plant is there by mistake, having evolved for hundreds of thousands of years to its current form. We may be missing out on great advances due to our lack of understanding when it comes to whole plants and herbs. When a plant shows benefits to humans, it's not just one isolated part that is doing all the work; you can be sure that every single component interacting with one another is contributing to the full scale benefits we receive.

Huge corporations are not operated just by the CEO; they have thousands and thousands of employees working together to run a successful company. And the United States government is not just operated by the president, but by the Senate, Congress, the executive branch, and the thousands of governmental employees who keep the system running. Just because the president seems more important than someone who works for the Environmental Protection Agency does not mean he or she alone creates the government. So why would we think that one ingredient in a plant is the full source of benefits for certain conditions? Seriously, who thought this was a good idea?

Instead of isolating what we think is the active ingredient, it's time to study all the compounds in the plant, and truly understand how they all interact. And while this may seem like the appropriate approach, there is pushback from the drug industry in a couple of forms. One, researching just one singular compound is way easier than researching multiple variants combined, and it's also easier to standardize a single compound into a drug. Two, manufacturing isolates is more profitable for pharmaceutical companies. You can patent single compounds and molecules, which could allow the drug company to profit upwards of billions of dollars. However, using the whole plant offers no such profitability. Plants don't tend to equal mad, mad money.

Using whole plant compounds also offers a safer approach—for example, consider the coca plant. We may know and recognize this plant for its birth of the harmful drug isolate cocaine, but what you probably don't know is that the coca leaf is one of the most beneficial plants out there. Andean Indians use the coca leaf more than any other medicine, specifically for constipation and diarrhea. When you look at the chemical constituents of the coca plant, you find there are fourteen active alkaloids, with the cocaine alkaloid being greatest in number. People may know that cocaine stimulates the gastrointestinal tract and makes bowels move more efficiently (I swear, I only know this from research), but when you take the whole plant with the fourteen other alkaloids, it can either stimulate the gut or inhibit the gut, depending on what your body needs. How amazing is that—a plant is able to change its course of action depending on what your specific needs are. But when you isolate out the cocaine alkaloid from the coca leaves, you get an addictive drug which makes people feel paranoid, hostile, angry, and anxious and can lead to a variety of consequences, including heart attack, permanent damage to the blood vessels of the heart and brain, tooth decay, malnutrition, psychosis, and depression.

This idea of using the whole versus its parts doesn't stop at just singular plants but also herbal formulations—for example, combining two or more herbs together for an even greater synergistic response. The potential for traditional herbal formulas to treat chronic conditions is astounding, but the potential for profits is lacking.

In no way is every condition appropriate for a whole herb intervention; however, when it comes to treating disease, it's important to look at a variety of approaches and not just the easier and more profitable ones. We could be missing out on some of the most exciting medical breakthroughs because we decided to take the easier route.

Herbs Deserve More Credit

Unpronounceable herbal remedies are more than just seasonings or added flavor to your turkey loaf; these substances are DNA-changing, immunity-boosting,

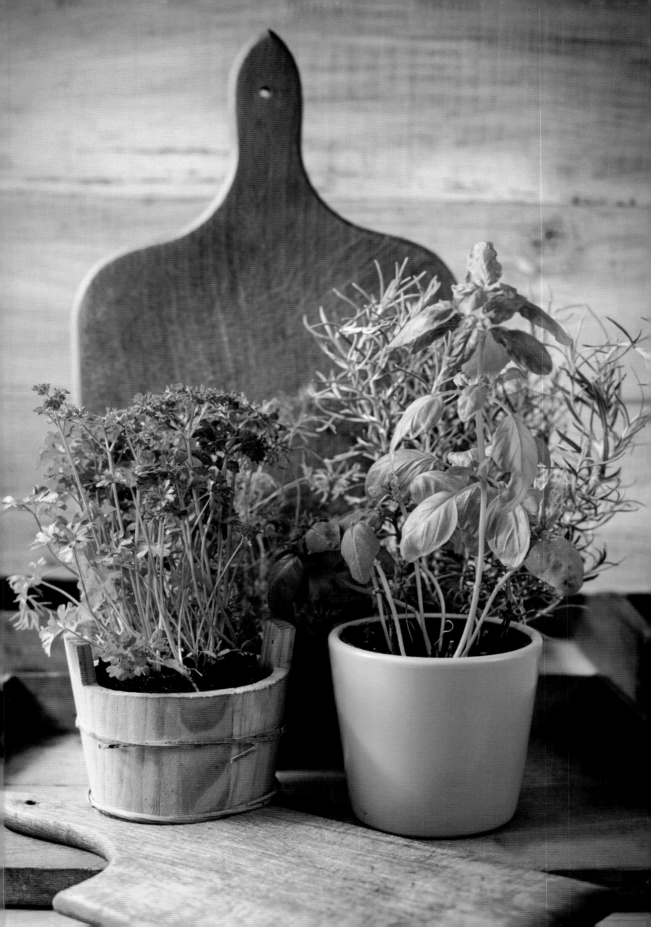

anti-inflammatory, cholesterol- and blood-pressure-lowering, anxiety-alleviating, stress-adapting, brain-bolstering, memory-enhancing, cancer-fighting, disease-preventing superplants.

With all the processed foods, inflammation, toxicity, sedentary lifestyles, stressful jobs, constant work, lack of play, and overmedication, of course our bodies are rebelling. And our illnesses are just our bodies' way of saying, "STOP! I need a break!"

With a change to our diets and lifestyle we can completely transform the way our body interacts and expresses itself. Health is a symptom of your body working. Illness is a symptom of unbalance. How many of us eat a diet of solely organic, local vegetables, fruits, and herbs, exercise and move our bodies on a regular and weekly basis, and sleep seven to nine hours per night, while taking time out

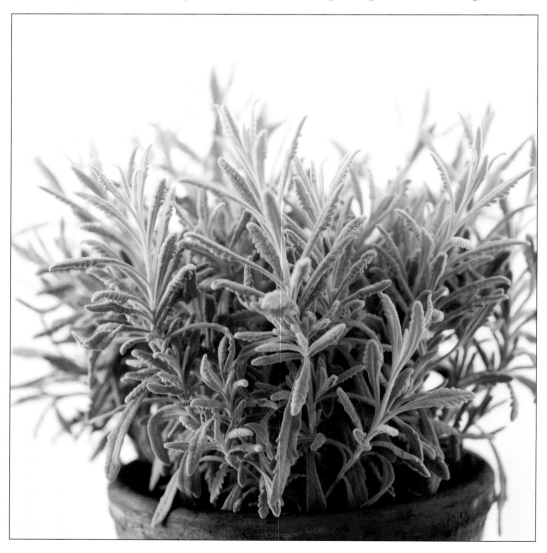

to socialize with friends and family, meditate, and make room to play and do what we love? Yes, adults need to play too. If this person exists, they're a dreamy unicorn, with undeniably good skin, and I want some of their magic.

While it may be extremely difficult to live the perfect unicorn lifestyle, there are tricks or hacks we can use to make us more prepared for our modern life, and some of these hacks include herbs. Tinctures, herbal formulas, homemade remedies, and other fun DIY herbal projects are a great way to propel your body back into balance. Herbs have been shown to reduce inflammation, promote blood flow, reduce tumor and cancer growth, lower blood sugar, reduce cholesterol, lower blood pressure, lower risk of heart disease, improve brain function, increase memory, delay the onset of Alzheimer's, positively change your gene expression, and more!

Plants basically turn you into a badass, superpowered, undercover health ninja. Who's in? Herbs obtain various chemical compounds as unpronounceable as polysaccharides, saponins, flavonoids, phytosterols, essential oils, micronutrients, antioxidants, thiosulfinates, anti-amyloids, polyphenols, and more. Herbs such as turmeric and ginger have become research darlings, with study after study showing the unbelievable health benefits associated with taking these medicinal plants on a regular basis. Who knew?

Well . . . herbalists knew.

But now the secret is out, and you are savvy to the immense healing benefits that herbs and plants have to offer. And with this book you will learn to make your own incredible herbal teas, scrubs, and formulas to help make your life a more healthful one. There's immense research out there confirming the health benefits of herbs and plant medicine, but why wait to use them? So get excited and start planting some amazing houseplants; you'll not only get fresher air and breathe in less toxins, but you'll also get a dose of anti-inflammatory, immune-boosting, health-promoting remedies that you can make inside your own home.

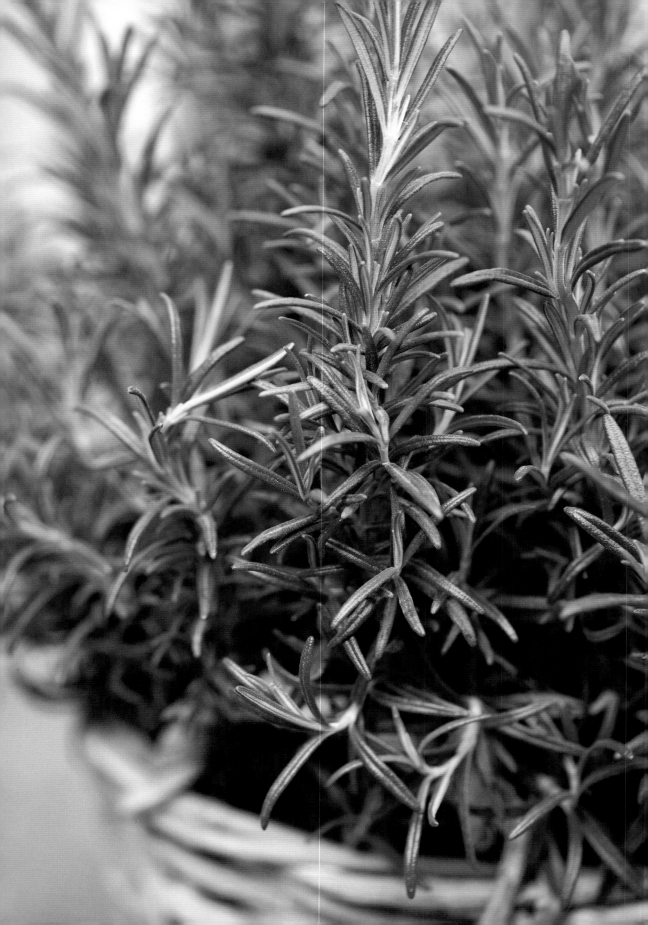

PART II

My Favorite Plants to Grow Indoors

"The healing comes from nature and not the physician. Therefore the physician must start from nature with an open mind."
—Paracelsus

"Nature itself is the best medicine."
—Hippocrates

"Flowers always make people better, happier, and more helpful; they are sunshine, food, and medicine to the soul."
—Luther Burbank

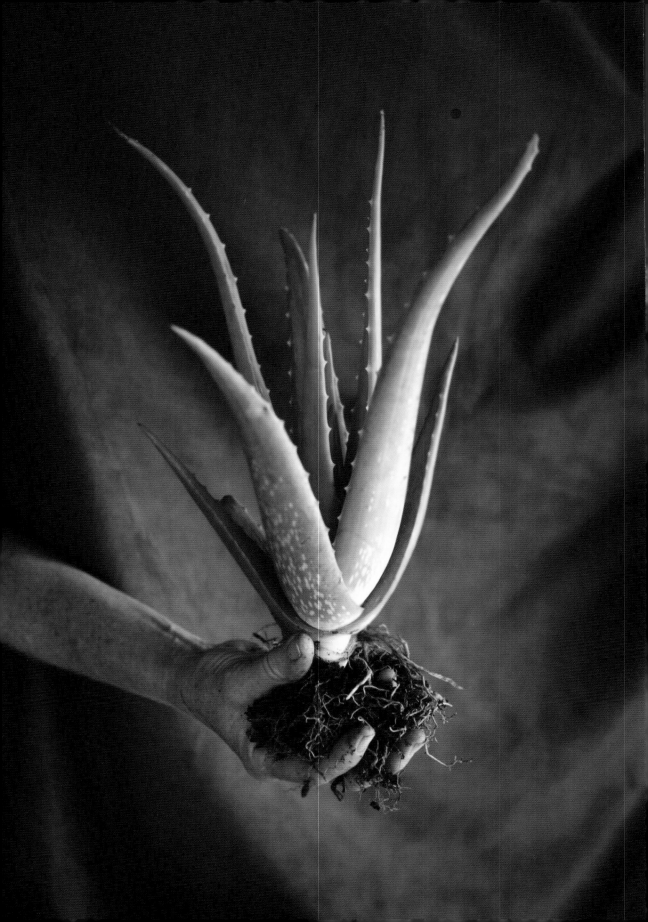

Chapter Three: Aloe Vera

Aloe barbadensis miller

Known as the "lily of the desert," "wonder plant," and more commonly the "burn plant," aloe vera, the spiky, green, desert-loving, alien-looking succulent originating from Africa is one of the easiest plants to keep alive and one of the most beneficial for your health. There are more than four hundred species of aloe, which can be grown indoors just about anywhere—I know you've seen one growing at your aunt Alice's house next to her terra-cotta sundial in Santa Fe. It can be found growing in the Southwest of the United States, Africa, Southeast Asia, Mexico, Central America, the West Indies, and the Bahamas.

Part of the succulent family, aloe is easy to care for, needs little water, has the ability to repair its own leaves, and is known for its capability to withstand a lot, including your neglect. Actually, aloe is so easy to care for that if you love neglecting plants, this is the one for you! A total win-win situation, a match made in heaven for you workaholics out there, it's time you got on the aloe train. Even more, if your cat decides to massacre your aloe plant by clawing it with its paws and causing the leaves to break, don't worry. Aloe will magically seal off the cut using its own gel and will continue to grow despite all the damage. Magic.

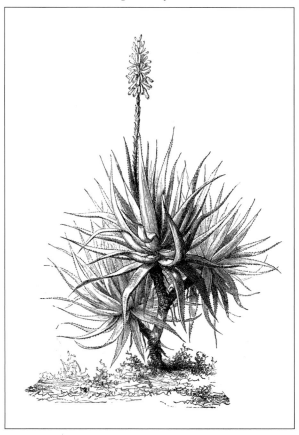

Aloe has been used medicinally for over six thousand years, dating back to early Egypt and depicted on stone carvings, and was known as the "plant of immortality" given as a gift to pharaohs at funeral processions. If aloe is good enough for pharaohs at funerals, it's good enough for you. History loves aloe, being documented from a Mesopotamian tablet, to ancient Egypt, to treating the soldiers who fought for Alexander the Great, to the Greeks, to modern-day *Baywatch*-loving sun worshippers. And for good reason. The aloe plant is a medicinal wonder, oozing out magical gel and containing a wonder juice that can be categorized as a superfood comprising a vast array of vitamins, minerals, and health-promoting agents. In fact, if you look all over the world, every traditional medicinal culture has found a way to use aloe in their medicines.

The Chinese use aloe for fungal infections and diseases, as well as promoting a healthy digestive system. Indonesians love aloe for their hair care; India uses it for constipation, infections, and skin diseases; Mexicans have used it to treat diabetes; and Americans love slathering it on their lobster bodies after a full day snoozing in the sun with a gin and tonic in their hand.

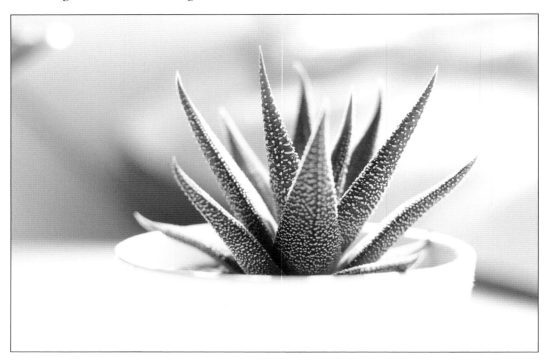

Getting to Know Your Aloe Vera Plant

Aloe is a spiky succulent, reminiscent of a cactus, with skinny, hard, slender leaves. If given the proper care, aloe can grow up to four feet tall and thrive indoors next to a window. These leaves contain a gel-like juice which contains a ton of nutrients.

Aloe has an amazing array of benefits and tons of uses, but it's important to understand the plant itself and its different properties. When growing, harvesting, and creating herbal remedies, you must learn and understand the whole plant and the many different qualities each part contains in order to properly harvest and safely obtain all the benefits.

For aloe, there are two main parts of the leaf that may be considered beneficial. These two parts are the gel, which is taken from the inner leaf, and the latex, which is the yellow oozing substance just under the skin of the leaf, or the outer leaf. While both portions of the leaf have uses, it is the inner leaf which contains most of the nutrients and health benefits. And it's the latex, or the outer leaf, which will have you running to the toilet, crying for your mom, regretting you ever knew the aloe plant existed in the first place.

INNER LEAF:

The most studied portion of the aloe plant, the inner leaf contains the aloe gel. When people incessantly talk about the health benefits of aloe, they are inevitably talking about the inner leaf and its oozing, translucent gel-like substance. Some of the benefits include supporting the immune system, supporting dental health, serving as an anti-inflammatory, and more.

OUTER LEAF/LATEX:

The outer leaf has what is known as the latex, the yellow juice near the rind. The latex contains aloin, which is not generally safe and has been shown to exacerbate Crohn's disease and ulcerative colitis, as well as deplete potassium and cause electrolyte imbalances, which may lead to muscle weakness and even cardiac problems. *Scary!* In 2002, the Food and Drug Administration (FDA) banned aloin from over-the-counter laxatives in the US. You should avoid any oral consumption of the aloin or aloe latex, as it can also cause kidney damage. Here's the most important lesson in herbalism: just because it's natural doesn't mean it's good for you.

So why would anyone use the latex to begin with? While mostly scary, there are a few benefits of the latex, but not enough for my taste. Used topically for skin irritations like sunburn, whole leaf extracts will contain parts of the outer leaf and can be beneficial. However, don't use on deep wounds, and be careful as some people have allergic reactions to the outer leaf. This usually only leads to a mild rash, but it's better to be safe than sorry. In general, the outer leaf should be avoided and discarded.

Buying Aloe Products

While this book is about creating your own herbal remedies, if you ever find yourself in a pinch and want to buy some aloe vera, here are a few tips. When buying aloe vera juice, gels, or lotions, look for products that only contain the inner portion of the leaf. These products will be anthraquinone or aloin (laxative) free. If you are buying lotions, look for the products with the highest percentage of the aloe gel.

Health Benefits

As with most plants, aloe contains a whole host of vitamins that the body needs, including A, C, E, B1, B2, B6, and B12. It also contains many minerals, such as calcium, sodium, iron, magnesium, potassium, and copper, but that's just to name a few. There are over seventy-five active components in aloe, including all the vitamins, minerals, amino acids, and organic compounds. It's pretty incredible what one spiky houseplant can do for your health.

Also found in aloe is a polysaccharide called acemannan which is known to have antiviral properties as well as ease gastrointestinal problems and boost the immune system. Aloe vera also has twenty amino acids, of which seven are essential fatty acids. There's a lot packed into the aloe vera plant, but how do these components translate to your health? What do they actually do for you?

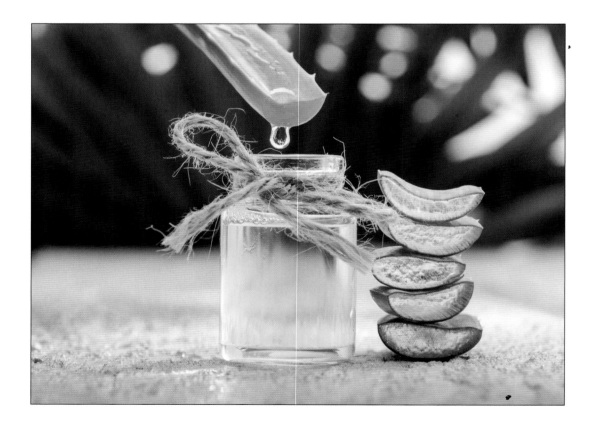

THE ULTIMATE SKIN REMEDY

We already know aloe's claim to fame of rehabilitating our chapped, burned, flaking, bodies after hours of basking in the sun—hello lobsters!—and for its ability to help heal irritations—hello rashes! When used topically, aloe gel is very effective as a treatment for a variety of skin conditions, not just the ones caused by our spring break in Cancun. The gel is able to help with a number of conditions, including cold sores, burns, abrasions, and psoriasis, of which there are three studies that show how effective aloe can be for mild psoriasis.

As a topical, it's been suggested as an effective treatment for first- and second-degree burns. Using aloe is no stranger to us; the FDA approved aloe vera ointment for skin burns in 1959, and we've all been lathering it on our bodies ever since. In fact, four studies found that aloe may reduce the healing time of burns by nine days compared to conventional treatments; however, when it comes to wound healing, studies are pretty inconclusive.[13]

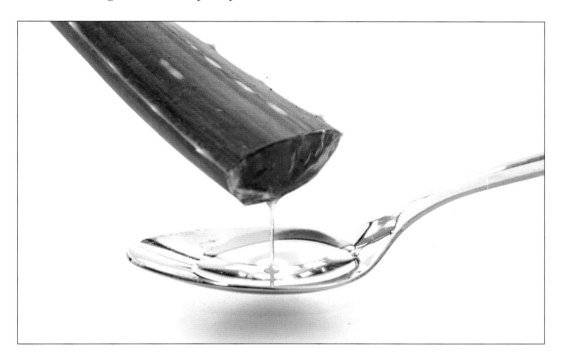

REDUCES DENTAL PLAQUE

You read that right, your teeth might benefit from the delightful oozing gel of aloe. A study found that those who used aloe vera juice as a mouthwash compared to those who use standard mouthwash found that after four days, aloe was found to be just as effective at reducing plaque as the standard products containing chlorhexidine.[14] The results were repeated in another study during a longer time period.[15] Apparently, aloe is able to kill plaque-friendly bacterium

Streptococcus mutans in the mouth as well as the yeast *Candida albicans*. Give me some aloe!

And if you are wondering why you would ever switch from your minty, delicious-tasting, last-minute toothpaste replacement mouthwash to gross aloe juice, here are some side effects of your standard mouthwash: brown staining of teeth, increased formation of tartar, oral dryness, that awful burning sensation you get while rinsing, and the inability to drink orange juice after rinsing away.

REDUCES CONSTIPATION

Aloe has been a remedy for constipation for thousands of years, with many traditional medicines using it as a main method to "float the boat." However, its laxative properties come from the outer portion of the leaf . . . yes, the scary latex is what causes you to run to the bathroom. If you need a laxative, it is probably best to use other sources to help.

ANTIAGING

If you want yet another product for your beauty regimen, why not try aloe! One very small study found that women over the age of forty-five who topically applied the gel to their face showed an increase in collagen production and improved skin elasticity over a ninety-day period.[16]

Collagen is found in our muscles, bones, tendons, skin, digestive system, and even our blood vessels. In fact, it's the most abundant protein in our body, and it helps our skin have elasticity and strength. Collagen helps build us, hold us together, and keeps us youthful. However, as we age our collagen production decreases and leads to wrinkles, sagging skin, chicken legs, and other qualities no one is waiting in line for. Supplementing with products that contain collagen, such as aloe, can help reduce the number of wrinkles and age better. Who doesn't want that?

ULCERS AND CANKER SORES NO MORE

Are you a canker sore person? What about mouth ulcers? These annoying reminders of pain are never welcome inside one's mouth and can last for over a week. A week of pain. However, some studies have shown that aloe may be a viable treatment for mouth ulcers and even speed up the healing process! It was found that an aloe vera patch applied to the area was effective at reducing the size of these unwelcome guests.[17] And a different study found that not only did the aloe speed up the healing process, but it also reduced pain levels.[18]

Possible Side Effects, Contraindications, and Drug Interactions

As with any herbal treatment, it's important to understand how it may interact with medications and drugs, or understand any possible side effects before you decide on treatment. In the case of aloe, as we've already mentioned, the latex of the plant should be avoided.

As with any plant, make sure you aren't allergic. If you are generally allergic to plants in the Liliaceae family, such as onions, garlic, and tulips, you should stay away. Otherwise, using the aloe gel topically is perfectly safe. People with diabetes should be careful ingesting aloe, as it can lower blood sugar.

If taking any medications, check to make sure yours doesn't interact with aloe. You can do this by going to the Mayo Clinic website.

Aloe Care Guide

Caring for aloe is famously easy. This is a great beginner houseplant, due to its general "chill" attitude and low number of needs. Aloe is the nonclingy girlfriend or boyfriend, who's comfortable enough to hang out by themselves at a party. They don't need a lot of attention. With that said, here are some instructions to care for your aloe plant.

Lighting: A plant that originates from Africa and thrives in all the hot, dry places in the world, it's no secret that aloe likes the sun. However, just because it loves the sun doesn't mean it can't be vulnerable with too much of it. In constant harsh light, aloe's leaves can turn brown, so make sure you give it bright, indirect light. In the winter, they've been known to freeze, so make sure you keep them away from any drafts or cold windows.

Water: Aloe does not like to stand in water, so make sure you are using well-draining soil, one that is made for cacti. Smaller pots will drain quickly, which would work better for this plant. Water sparingly, once per week or longer, and let the soil dry out between watering.

Troubleshooting Aloe:

Q: What if my leaves are lying flat?
A: Not to worry. If the leaves look depressed and flat, this is most likely due to a lack of light. Place the aloe in a window where it's sure to get some sunshine, and you'll see the leaves bounce back.

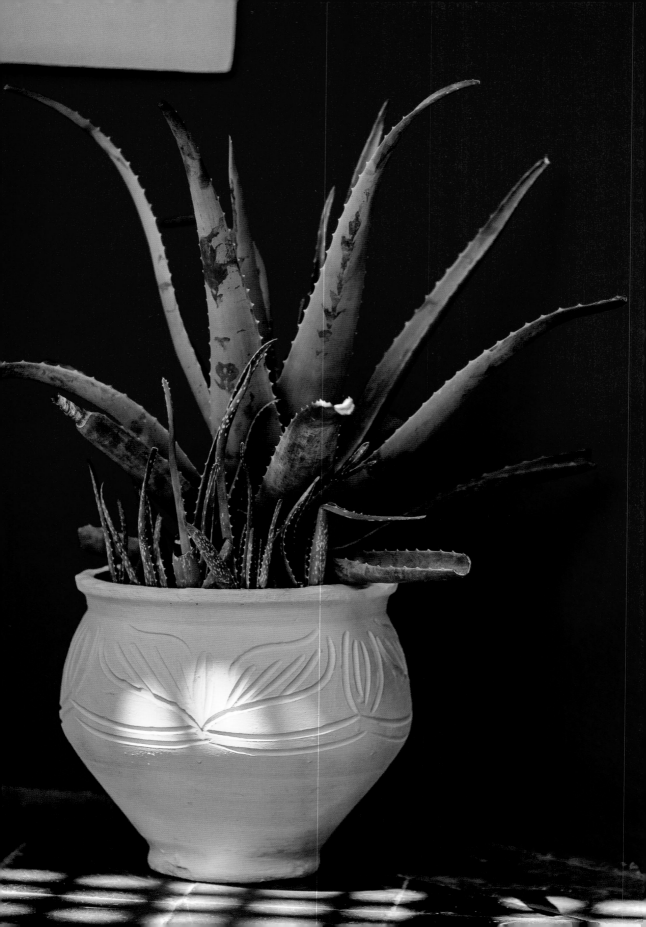

Q: Why are my leaves thin and curled?
A: This sounds like a classic case of underwatering!

Q: Why are my leaves brown?
A: This all depends on what kind of brown they resemble. If the leaves are brown and limp, it could be a sign of overwatering. If they are brown at the tips, or spotted along the leaves it could be due to overexposure to the sun. Yes, plants can burn too! When aloe gets too much sun, its symptoms may resemble those of typical sunburns and will become dry and brown. Take your plant to a less bright location, and see if this helps.

Recipes and Remedies

This is the part you've probably been waiting for: it's finally time to start making cool, useful, exciting homemade remedies from your aloe! There are vast amounts of information for aloe when it comes to making great DIY remedies; there are so many options when it comes to aloe gel. Below are a few of my favorite recipes, and I'm so excited to share them with you.

First, I want to show you how to harvest the all-important gel from its leaves. This is an easy process, though you might get sticky.

HARVESTING ALOE GEL

1. Cut out the thickest, largest leaf you can find. If possible, make sure the plant is mature enough; look for the leaves with a nice rose hue, and avoid the smaller leaves—they're still growing. Don't worry about taking a leaf; the plant will grow back, but make sure not to take too many at once. You don't want to leave it barren and lonely.
2. Take out your favorite sharp and clean knife and cut the leaf off as close to the trunk of the plant as possible.
3. Make sure to hold the end with the cut edge down so you can allow the yellow latex to drip out—this may take upwards of thirty minutes. Remember, we don't want that nasty stuff.
4. Cut off the spiky, serrated edges.
5. Filet the leaf like a fish until you have two pieces of the aloe leaf. Take a spoon and scrape out the translucent gel—this is the best part, very therapeutic! Place the gel into your mason jar to save for later use.

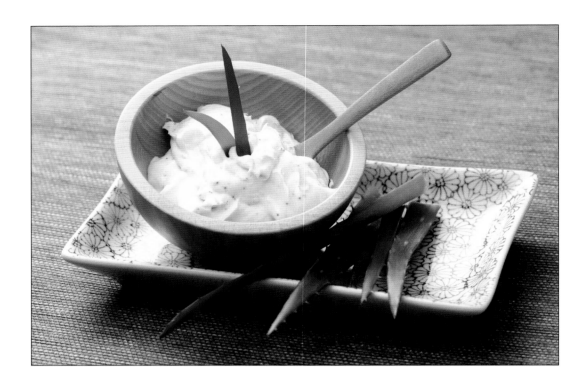

Aloe Vera Face Cream

We can't talk about aloe without create an amazing face remedy with its amazing gel. By harvesting your own aloe gel, you are skipping out on all the additives, preservatives, and other unpronounceable additions to your store-bought aloe. With this recipe, you are getting pure, nature-made, skin-loving cream, plus the bragging rights to all your friends and family that you are "*so* DIY."

Ingredients:

- Aloe gel from a small leaf
- ½ cup extra-virgin coconut oil
- A few drops essential oil of your choice (I prefer geranium, lavender, and ylang-ylang)

Instructions:

1. Take the gel from your small aloe leaf and place it in a blender. Blend the gel until it's light and frothy.
2. Place your blended aloe gel and ½ cup coconut oil into a bowl and whisk the two together using an electric hand blender for about five minutes until you get a consistency that's light, like a cake frosting.

3. Add a few drops of your choice of essential oil. I like using lavender because it's great for the skin, can help heal irritations, and the scent is relaxing and calming. Geranium is a wonderful oil, which can balance oil production and condition the skin, and is a great addition to moisturizers. Ylang-ylang is a great oil to help treat acne and oily skin, and may help fight the effects of aging by stimulating cell growth! If you're feeling extra saucy, why not add a drop of each to the cream! I have no idea how that will end up smelling, but I'm excited to hear about your experience.

4. Whisk the oil again with your potpourri of essential oils. After you're done, place your lotion into a glass container and store it in the refrigerator. You can use this anywhere on your body, in the morning, after a shower, before bed, when you're bored, literally whenever you want! The lotion should last for several weeks in your fridge, so make sure to use it before it expires.

Don't Use Sparingly

This gooey mixture is wonderful for your skin as it puts together two of the most skin-loving ingredients: coconut oil and aloe gel. Coconut oil is known for its antibacterial and antifungal properties, is an amazing and tropical-smelling moisturizer, and actually penetrates your skin on a deeper level than most other oils—this is due to its low molecular weight and how it bonds with proteins (science!). With that said, coconut oil can help reduce bacterial infections on the skin and help prevent acne breakouts; it's also a great protection from the sun, naturally providing you with a sun protection factor of four. This stuff is amazing; too bad it doesn't come from a houseplant. The mix of coconut oil with aloe gives you a moisturizing kick in the butt, helps you look younger, and makes you smell like the Garden of Eden. And remember, don't use sparingly. Slather this on your body like you're about to enter a mud wrestling match. Your skin will thank you later.

Aloe Vera Hand Sanitizer

Forget the countless antibacterial hand sanitizers out there; if you've learned anything from this book thus far, it's that we overuse these little bottles of bacteria killers. So if you want to be an agent of change against the antibiotic crisis, while at the same time having clean hands, why not make your own hand sanitizer with aloe and essential oils. This is an easy way to help clean your hands, but it won't contribute to the mess that's happening worldwide with our overuse of antibacterial *everything*.

Ingredients:

- 8 ounces aloe gel
- 10 drops lavender essential oil
- 30 drops tea tree oil
- ¼ teaspoon vitamin E oil
- 1 tablespoon high-proof vodka

Instructions:

1. Place your aloe gel in the blender until it's light and frothy. Combine the essential oils and vitamin E oil in a small glass bowl and mix.
2. Add the alcohol to the oils and blend again.
3. Finally, add the aloe vera gel and mix well. Place in a dark glass spritzer bottle and shake gently before each use.

Incredibly Simple Aloe Burn Cream

We've all done it: burned ourselves while cooking, lighting a match, or just playing with fire (not recommended). But when we find ourselves burned or scraped, aloe is a great remedy to have on hand. This simple remedy will be your go-to burn treatment and help you heal faster and with less pain.

Ingredients:

- 1 aloe vera leaf
- 1 teaspoon vitamin E oil

Instructions

1. Trim a leaf using a diagonal cut. Peel one side of the leaf with a vegetable peeler. Start at the top and work your way down.
2. Let the yellow liquid drain out first and discard. Use a spoon to scrape out the translucent part of the aloe plant and add to a blender. Mix in the vitamin E oil and puree the mixture.
3. Rub on your burns or scrapes for faster healing!

This incredibly easy recipe uses the antibacterial properties of tea tree oil and lavender oil. The added alcohol will help preserve the mixture, together with the vitamin E oil. This recipe is a great alternative to the chemical sanitizers used widely today. Essential oils are able to provide antibacterial properties, but they don't add to the problem of bacterial resistance like chemical cleansers. Again, nature tends to find a balance, and essential oils are being seen as one of the many options to help combat bacterial antibiotic resistance, due to their complex chemical makeup and ability to work synergistically.

Aloe vera is everyone's beginner plant; placed on the windowsill and often forgotten, it still manages to thrive in everyone's neglect. With aloe's unique aesthetic of the desert, reminiscent of the cacti populating those surroundings, who doesn't love the look of it and other indoor succulents for their decor? When I was a struggling gardener, aloe was one of my first successes. It allowed me to practice my green thumb skills, forgiving me for too much water or too little, too much sun or not enough. Not to mention, aloe gave me the healing gel for my various kitchen burns when I was (and still am) learning to cook. I think everyone should have an aloe plant in their lives, not only for their good looks, cleaner air, and loving, healing gel, but also for the fact that they refuse to die. We all need that kind of perseverance in our lives.

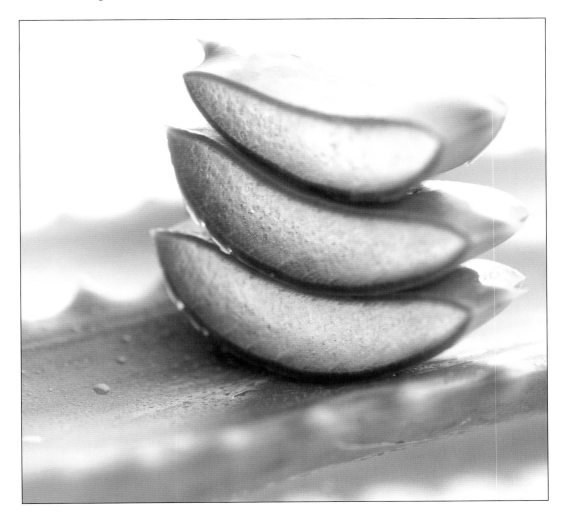

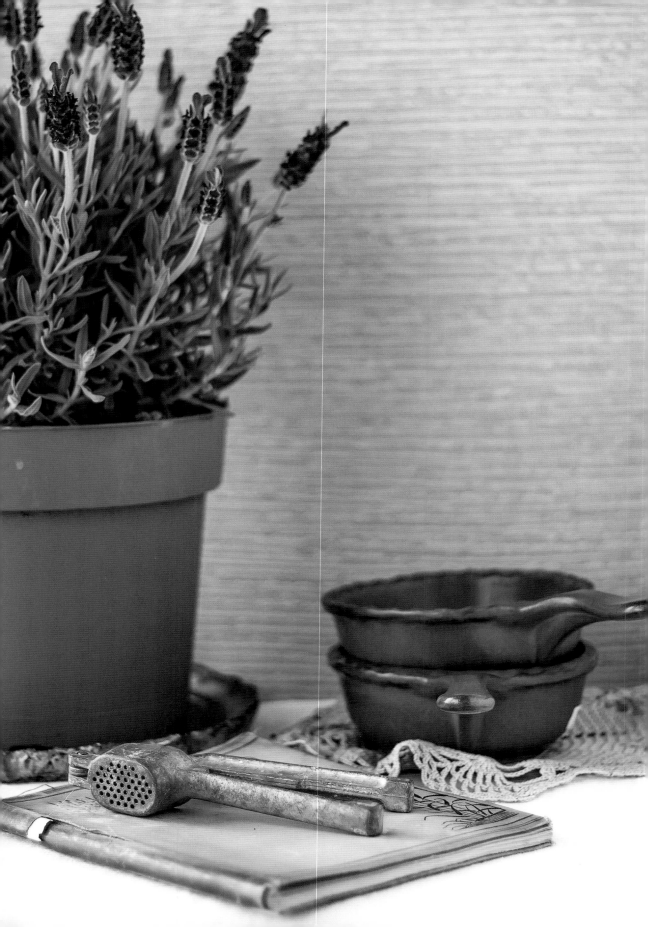

Chapter Four: Lavender

Lavendula

One of the most popular herbs on earth, lavender can be found in almost every bath salt, calming cream, essential oil, or overpriced spa treatment. To many, relaxation doesn't begin until the scent of lavender wafts into their nose after rubbing lavender-scented lotion on their hands, lighting their boutique lavender candles, and sitting in an elegant Jacuzzi bath with lavender essential oil while listening to Kenny G. Yes, lavender may be the king of calm, but it's so much more.

With over twenty different species, lavender is actually in the mint family and has been historically used for over 2,500 years. This sweet-smelling flowering plant originates from the Middle East and Mediterranean, and has been used by the Greeks, Syrians, Romans, Egyptians, and all throughout antiquity.

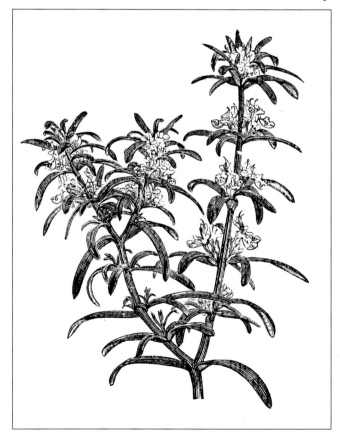

The word lavender comes from the Latin word *lavare*, which means "to wash," and it's stayed true to its name. Lavender was used as an ingredient in herbal baths by the Romans and Greeks; the ancient Egyptians used it as a perfume (just like when you want to mask the fact you haven't showered in two days), mummification, and an ingredient for incense. During the Middle Ages it was used as an aphrodisiac often considered as the "herb of love." It's also been used as a disinfectant for castles and sick rooms, and as a wound cleaner during wartime. Lavender has been used for almost everything from a delicious culinary spice to embalming corpses. And it's still used just as widely today, for almost as many varied reasons—maybe not the embalming, though.

In our modern era, lavender was "rediscovered" when aromatherapist René Gattefossé burned his hand and used lavender to help it heal. He verified lavender's healing and antiseptic qualities when the plant's oils helped stop the pain almost immediately and no infection, scarring, inflammation, or redness occurred.

Today, lavender is grown throughout the world, from the US to New Zealand, Canada, Australia, Japan, Spain, the Netherlands, and more. However, nothing beats Provence, France, when it comes to quantity. Provence has been growing lavender for centuries, passing down the herbal growing tradition in families from generation to generation. And while the initial demand for lavender was a slow build, business started growing in the beginning of the twentieth century when lavender oils started becoming more and more popular. To this day, Provence is the number-one producer of lavender, with fields upon fields of beautiful purple hues winding up and down hills and valleys during the peak months of June through early August.

Health Benefits

Like most herbs, lavender has a wide array of health benefits and medicinal uses, including relieving anxiety and stress, helping heal burns and wounds, reducing

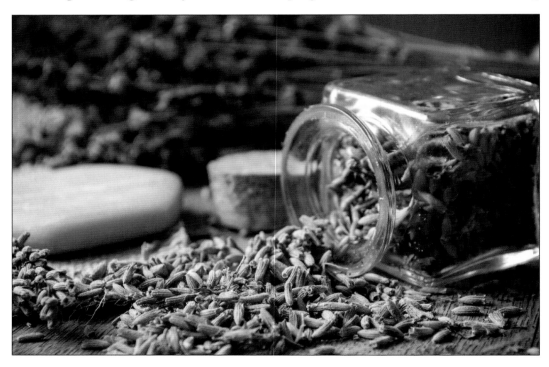

acne and clearing up the skin, improving sleep, calming the mind, alleviating headaches, and more. And these benefits aren't just anecdotal; research is proving that lavender is a powerful healer.

HEALS CUTS AND WOUNDS

As mentioned earlier, lavender has quite the history of healing cuts and wounds, and I'm not just talking about little scrapes and bruises you got while trying to rollerblade for the first time outside of your kitchen floor. During World War I, lavender oil was used as an antiseptic and disinfectant to help treat soldiers' wounds and sterilize the medical equipment. We can all remember how aromatherapist René Gattefossé helped heal his own burns using the essential oil topically—he noticed a great reduction in pain and faster healing.

There are more than one hundred studies which confirm these historical uses, showing that lavender speeds up healing of cuts and burns due to its antimicrobial properties. One study found that lavender is able to boost collagen synthesis, thus promoting the body to repair itself, promoting the formation of new scar tissue, and healing faster.[19]

And when mixed together with other oils, it can speed up the healing process even faster. It's been shown that lavender's antimicrobial effects are enhanced when mixed together with oils like cinnamon, tea tree, or clove. Talk about synergistic effects—this is the basis of herbalism.

BENEFITS THE SKIN

We already know that lavender oil is great for cuts and wounds, but what about other maladies of the skin? With amazing antimicrobial and antioxidant capabilities, lavender works great for acne, eczema, and psoriasis, working to help reduce the inflammation, inhibiting the bacterial formation that causes acne in the first place, helping regulate hormones which cause acne during your period, and helping previous acne scars to heal and reduce.

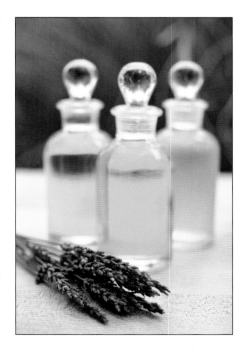

Researchers in Portugal found that pathogenic skin strains hate lavender oil, as it killed a host of pathogenic fungi, killing the fungal cell's membrane. Lavender is potent medicine to help fight fungal infections, especially those on the skin, so if you're sick and tired of dealing with your acne to no end, why not try lavender?

ANXIETY AND STRESS

You can't walk into a spa or healing center without smelling the intense floral aromas of lavender upon entering. Lavender is associated with calm, turning you from a screaming monster in traffic into a zen meditating master. And while lavender can seem overused these days, it's for good reason. It works.

More than 6.8 million adults suffer from anxiety in the United States, and even more suffer from daily stress. And while many will turn to medications such as Xanax or Valium, why not first try herbs such as lavender? Lavender has been shown to be an effective powerhouse when it comes to treating anxiety, and without all the side effects of pharmaceutical interventions.

For example, in a study published in the journal *Phytomedicine*, it was found that lavender oil was as effective as the drug lorazepam (Ativan) in treating signs of anxiety, but it didn't make patients feel fatigued and has no potential for drug abuse.[20] More research has shown lavender to help with nervousness, restlessness, and symptoms of depression, and it can also help people who suffer from agitation related to dementia.

A different study in the *International Journal of Psychiatry in Clinical Practice* found that taking 80-mg capsules of lavender essential oil helps alleviate depression and anxiety and leads to better sleep[21]. But you don't have to ingest it to get great results; just diffusing lavender oil at home can lead to a reduction in postnatal depression and a decrease in anxiety symptoms after four weeks of using the essential oil diffuser.

Anxiety can be overwhelming and stress inducing, leading you into a cycle of stress leading to anxiety, leading to more stress, and on and on and on, oh joy! However, the good news is that there are options, and not all of them have to have scary side effects. Lavender not only smells good but is a potent medicinal proven to help calm the mind and lower your stress levels. Not to mention, it smells like spa day.

PREMENSTRUAL SYNDROME

Talk to any woman and she'll surely tell you how she wished her premenstrual syndrome (PMS) symptoms would just go away. PMS might be the butt of many jokes, but in reality it's not so much fun. These symptoms occur around one week (or more) before a woman's menstruation and are related to hormone changes due to her cycle.

An estimated 85 percent of women suffer from some sort of PMS, which can include many fun symptoms, such as breast tenderness, irritability, anxiety,

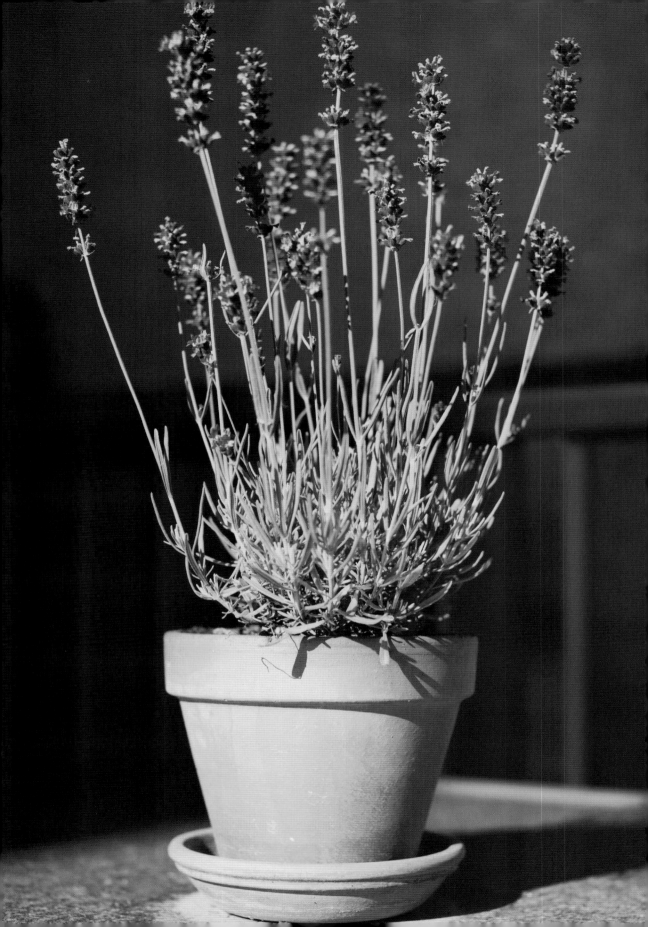

mood swings, depression, appetite changes, joint pain, cramping, fatigue, bloating, headaches or migraines, acne, nausea, and digestive changes.[22] Luckily, most women don't experience all those symptoms because that would just be cruel.

Hormone balance is crucial to having a seamless period and cycle, and luckily lavender has been shown to balance these hormones and alleviate many of the major premenstrual symptoms. Lavender can also alleviate feelings of stress, depression, or anxiety before menstruation. It can also specifically aid in sometimes inexplicable changes in emotions, like sobbing during a car commercial—inhaling lavender oil has been shown to decrease these symptoms after just ten minutes.[23]

INSOMNIA

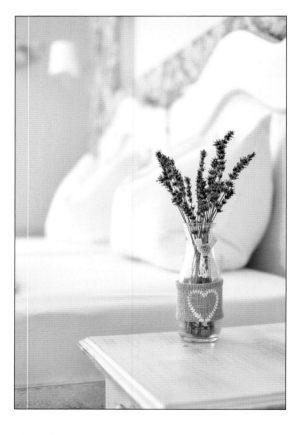

Without sleep, we can't function. A normal day at work turns into a marathon of trying to keep your head from hitting the table and drool dripping down your chin. And Americans have trouble sleeping. More than 30 percent of Americans suffer from insomnia, and more than half of Americans lose sleep to anxiety and stress. That's a lot of restless nights. Luckily, lavender can help in two ways: reducing your stress and anxiety and helping your mind drift off into la-la land.

There is a lot of research that shows the effectiveness of lavender on your sleep cycle. One such study from psychologists at Wesleyan University asked thirty-one men and women to sniff lavender essential oil one night and then sniff plain, diffused water the next night for two-minute periods before bed. What they found was that the lavender oil was effective in helping the participants sleep more soundly and wake up with more energy[24]. Yes, this is a very small study, but the results are promising for future research. The researchers also found that the reason why lavender might be useful in helping you sleep may be how it's able to increase slow-wave sleep—this is the sleep where your muscles relax, your heartbeat slows down, and your memories are organized.

More small studies have corroborated this evidence, showing lavender to be useful for slumbering. It's been shown to help geriatric patients who have recently stopped benzodiazepine treatment regain their sleep. Unexpectedly, when these patients went off their drugs, sleep patterns were disturbed. However, it was found that using lavender oil aromatherapy was able to restore the patient's sleep back to levels similar to those when they were on benzodiazepines.[25] Not too shabby for a plant.

HEADACHES

If you are unlucky enough to suffer from migraines and nasty headaches, lavender might be just what the doctor ordered. Recent research has shown that lavender may be a safe and effective treatment for those awful migraines. Headaches have all sorts of triggers, be they hormonal, stress, allergic reactions, and so on. If you're a woman, chances are hormonal fluctuations of estrogen may be the cause of the pain, especially before your period, not to mention the fluctuations of hormones during menopause (fun!). With that in mind, lavender is a great natural way to balance hormones and help relieve and prevent headaches around your cycle. Even better, if your headaches are caused by stress, there is nothing like lavender to relieve you of your suffering! It's also an amazing stress remedy, keeping you calm during rush hour traffic or, worse, when you run out of Nutella.

Possible Side Effects, Contraindications, and Drug Interactions

Lavender oil is toxic when taken orally. Pregnant and breastfeeding women should avoid using lavender. Some people may develop an allergic reaction, causing nausea, vomiting, headache, and chills. It may also cause skin irritation when applied directly to the skin.

There are no known scientific reports of interactions between lavender and common medications. However, possible interactions with central nervous system (CNS) depressants may occur, as lavender promotes relaxation. This may make the depressants even stronger. Such drugs include morphine or oxycodone, Ativan, Valium, and Xanax.

Lavender Care Guide

Lavender is an amazing plant to grow indoors, making your home smell like a fresh field in Provence, or a DIY spa. However, lavender can be tricky to grow indoors, so bring some patience and excitement to this endeavor. First, it's important to choose the right kind of lavender for your home, and in this case French lavender should do the trick; even though it won't have the strongest aroma, it will have the best chance for survival in your home.

Lighting: Lavender needs lots of light, so if you happen to live in the basement (I'm talking to all the "garden unit" dwellers) it might not be such a good idea to grow lavender. Place your plant in the sunniest part of your home; if you aren't lucky enough to have a light-filled house, make sure to get some grow lights or broad spectrum plant lights. And don't forget to rotate your plant every few days to allow every part to get its sunshine.

Water: Always allow the soil to dry out in between watering; you don't want to overwater. Lavender hates feeling moist and soggy, so make sure to let it dry out. Soil should be dry to the touch.

Soil: Use well-drained soils that are slightly alkaline.

Temperature: Don't let your lavender sit next to any drafts or cold air. When the weather starts getting warm outside, put your lavender plant out in the sunshine. This will help your plant mature and encourage growth. When everything is said and done, you'll notice that your lavender blooms will peak from late June through August.

Pruning: Pruning your lavender depends on the type you're trying to grow. The most commonly grown lavender, English lavender, should be pruned in late August, cutting it back by two thirds. You should notice new growths appearing shortly, becoming hardy before the approaching winter.

Recipes and Remedies

Now that you have a healthy, beautiful lavender plant to show off to all your friends, let's take it one step further and create some amazing remedies you can use every day for your health, wellness, and just plain bragging rights.

Lavender Oil

Lavender oil will be one of the most useful homemade medicinals you have in your home—its uses are wide and varied. From skincare to baths, soaps, and lotions, lavender oil will be the "why not?" product you have in your cabinet. Not to mention, it smells amazing.

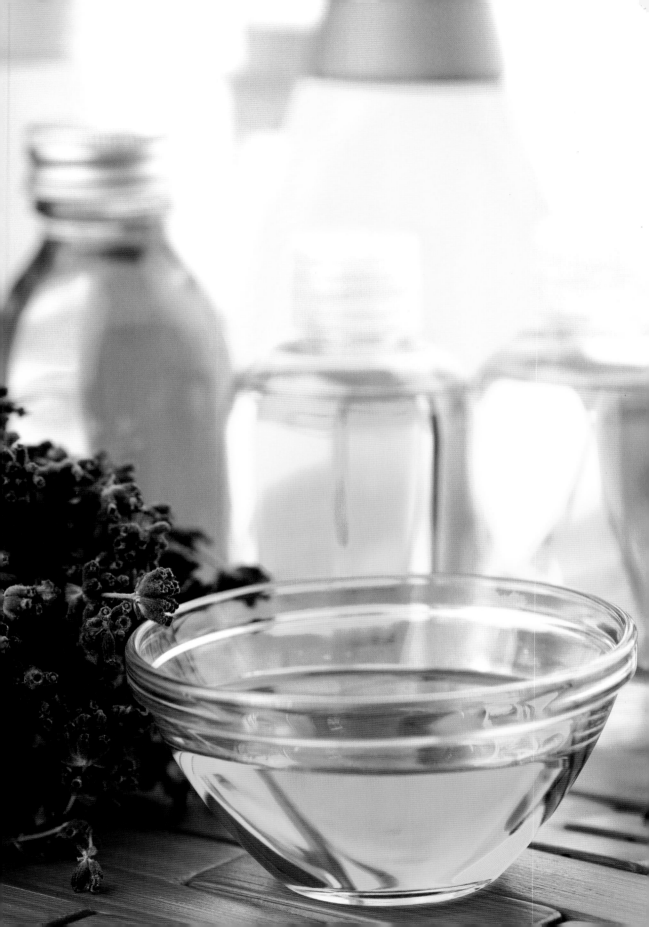

Ingredients:

- Fresh lavender flowers just about to open
- Mason jar
- Base oil, such as sweet almond oil or olive oil
- Paper bag
- Glass bottle
- Cheesecloth

Instructions:

1. Pick lavender flowers just before they're about to open and place them in a sterile, dry, and clean mason jar.
2. Cover the flowers completely with your choice of base oil. Make sure no parts of the flowers are sticking out; this could lead to mold.
3. Cover with a lid, place the jar in a paper bag, and leave it near a sunny window for about two weeks.
4. After about two weeks, decant the liquid into a glass bottle, using a cheesecloth to separate out the flowers and plant parts from the oil.

Your oil is now ready to use, on its own, or in another recipe. Combine with other oils, use on your skin as a moisturizer (to avoid skin irritation, mix the oil with a carrier such as coconut oil), place it in bath salts, or just take a sniff every day. Lavender oil can and should be used widely in your home. Plus, it's so easy to make, there's no excuse!

Lavender Balm

Lavender balm is a great way to preserve lavender oil and turn it into a topical anti-inflammatory. Use it on sore muscles, dry hands and feet, along your temples, or anywhere you are in pain. The mixture of lavender oil with vitamin E oil and almond oil will give your body an anti-inflammatory head start, allowing your body to relax and begin to heal.

Ingredients:

- 40 grams shea butter
- 18 grams beeswax
- 110 grams sweet almond oil
- 3 drops Vitamin E oil
- ¼ teaspoon lavender oil

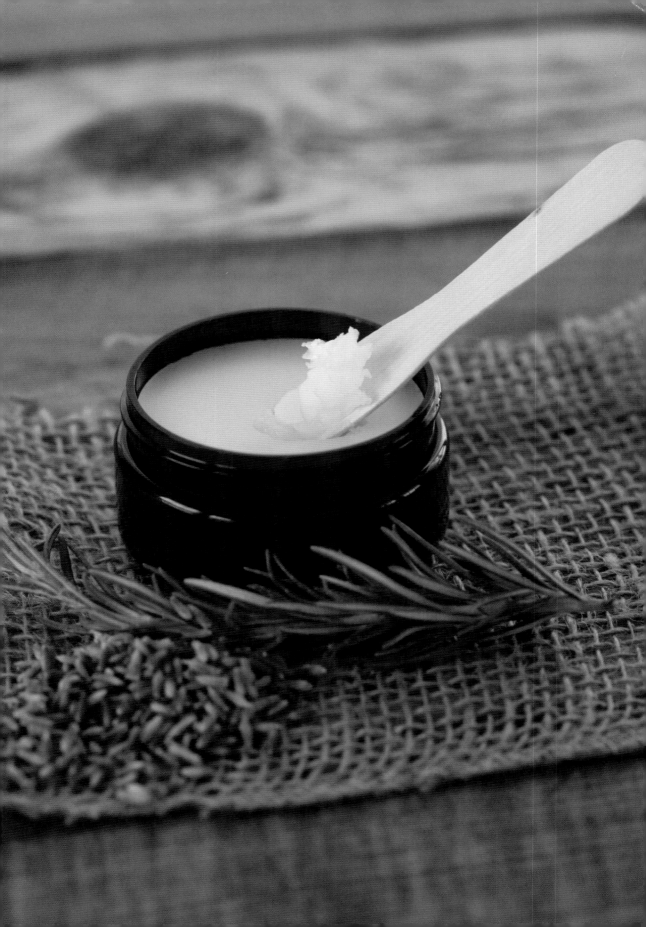

Instructions:

1. Over low heat, melt the shea butter and beeswax until they are a liquid. Once they are liquid, add the sweet almond oil.
2. Take the oils off the heat and allow them to sit until the temperature is below 130°F or 54°C. Once the oils are just below 130°F, mix in the vitamin E and lavender oil and pour the concoction evenly into containers.
3. You should allow the balm to cool for thirty minutes before you move it, and don't place a lid on it until the balm is cool and hardened.

You can use these handy balms for up to two years, but it's always best to use it as soon as possible.

Lavender Bath Salt

Bath salts are a wonderful way to relax and unwind after a long day, not to mention they're incredible for your muscles. In fact, Epsom salts are known to be high in magnesium and to be a natural anti-inflammatory. Many athletes soak in Epsom salts after a hard workout, and the benefits don't stop there. By some estimates, up to 80 percent of people are deficient in magnesium, a mineral necessary for regulating over three hundred enzymes in the body, aiding in the detoxification process, and repairing your DNA![26] This is no small task.

Simply soaking in a Epsom salts bath will bring your magnesium levels up, and eventually bring you out of a deficiency. The magnesium in the salts not only helps with sore muscles, but it is known to reduce stress and calm the mind. In fact, research out of the University of North Carolina has found that low levels of magnesium increase stress reactions and have a huge effect on neural excitability.[27] If you are low on magnesium, chances are you are feeling stressed or agitated, or even suffering from panic attacks. But that's not all; deficiency signs also include tingling and numbness, fatigue, muscle cramps and contractions, depression, hypertension, and more. Luckily, salt baths are a great way to increase your magnesium levels and lead you back to normal.

And if you are someone who enjoys a good detox, look no further than your bath salts. Forget starving yourself while drinking a gross mixture of lemon, cayenne, and maple syrup; just take a bath! The sulfates found in Epsom salts help the body flush out toxins and provide a heavy metal detox. The salts are able to trigger a process called reverse osmosis, pulling salt out of your body along with all the nasty toxins.

The mix of Epsom salts and lavender will give you a relaxing combo, allowing your mind to rest, your muscles to relax, and your body to detox.

Ingredients:

- ¾ cup Epsom salts
- ½ cup Dead Sea salt
- 2 tablespoons dried lavender buds
- 1 tablespoon safflower oil
- ⅛ teaspoon vitamin E oil
- 8 to 10 drops lavender essential oil

Instructions:

Combine all your ingredients in a bowl and mix well. Place your mixture in an airtight container, preferably glass. Let the mixture sit for several days so the essential oils and fresh herbs can infuse into the salts. That's it! Pour the salts into a hot tub for a restorative soak.

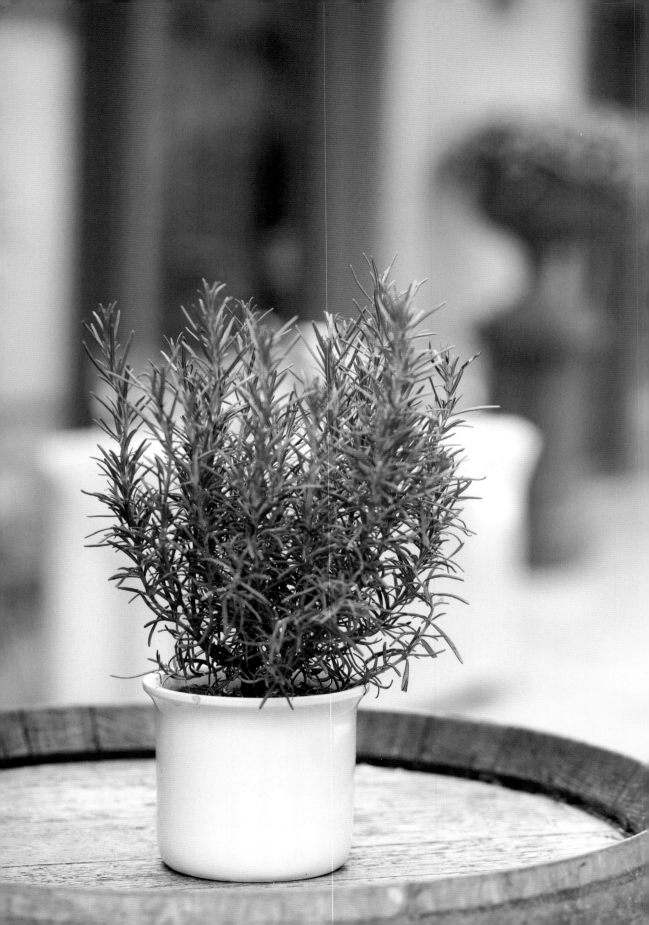

Chapter Five: Rosemary

Rosmarinus officinalis

Often thought of as a culinary herb, rosemary is more than just a garnish, and despite its name, rosemary has nothing to do with roses or a woman named Mary. Actually, the name stems from the Latin word *rosmarinus*, which means "dew of the sea," a reference to its light-blue flowers and love for wet environments.

A member of the mint family, rosemary has been traditionally used in Mediterranean cuisine; you might recognize it doused in olive oil, sprinkled over chicken, and eventually lodged in between your two front teeth. Its anti-inflammatory effects and antioxidant properties promote health and wellness and provide many health benefits, which include improving digestion, helping prevent hair loss, reducing skin irritations, enhancing memory, promoting eye health, and perhaps even preventing brain aging.

Recorded uses of rosemary date back to 500 BC, when it was used by the ancient Romans and Greeks for its medicinal, culinary, and mystical properties. Roman gardens almost always had rosemary bushes, and many believed they grew only in the gardens of those who were righteous, while protecting people from evil spirits. Today, we also use rosemary as a means to protect us, but for health purposes rather than evil ghosts.

If you're a fan of English literature, Shakespeare's Juliet was buried with rosemary as an honor of her remembrance—many early Europeans were buried with sprigs of rosemary as a symbol that the dead would not be forgotten. To this day rosemary is used as a funeral flower, symbolizing remembrance and respect for those who had passed. But death isn't rosemary's only claim to fame; love and romance often look to rosemary as a fixture in weddings, courtships, and fidelity. However, I don't believe bringing home a sprig of rosemary would do much today to swoon your beloved. Although maybe a potted rosemary plant would!

Health Benefits

Rosemary's unique past shows the importance of this culinary herb often overlooked not only in culture and tradition but also for its healing properties. When eating your favorite Mediterranean dishes you might not be aware that the rosemary garnish is a good source of calcium, iron, potassium, magnesium, manganese, and vitamin B6, and recent research has discovered many potential health benefits related to memory and concentration, preventing hair loss, reducing stress, and improving digestion, just to name a few. After learning about the various health benefits of this herbal sprig, rosemary will never look or taste the same again.

IMPROVES DIGESTION

Approved for the treatment of digestion by Germany's Commission E, rosemary is used by many Europeans as a digestive aid, although there isn't a lot of scientific evidence to support this claim. It's important to note, however, that research has a long way to catch up with herbal medicine and that shouldn't stop you from safely using herbs to improve your life and health. Thousands of years of tradition and anecdotal evidence should be noted. In this case, rosemary has a lot of history for its use in digestion, such as helping reduce gas, upset stomach, and indigestion.

IMPROVES MEMORY AND CONCENTRATION

For thousands of years, one of the most popular uses for rosemary has been to improve memory. The Greeks would place rosemary sprigs in their hair while studying for tests, and it was often used as an aromatherapy for cognitive decline due to aging. Research from *Therapeutic Advances in Psychopharmacology*

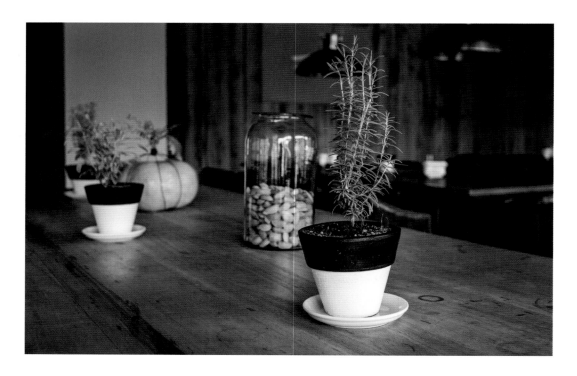

has found that the aroma of rosemary essential oil affects cognition and improves a person's concentration, accuracy, mood, and performance.[28] Try it next time when you have a big meeting or need to study for a big exam—make sure to study with a few drops of the essential oil on your temples and wrists. The aroma of rosemary will trigger your memory recall and help you ace those big moments.

A different study tested the effects of rosemary on cognitive function in an elderly population and found that rosemary essential oil had a significant improvement on their performance and overall memory and improved the speed of retrieving memories. In fact, speed of memory is a predictor of cognitive function during aging, and rosemary was found to have a statistically significant effect.[29]

FIGHTS CANCER

Numerous studies have found that rosemary can play a role in preventing cancers such as colorectal, breast, and ovarian. Rosemary extract contains numerous polyphenols, such as carnosic acid, carnosol, and rosmarinic acid, all of which inhibit the proliferation of certain cancer cell lines.[30]

A study published in *Bioscience, Biotechnology, and Biochemistry* found that rosemary is also useful as an antitumor agent.[31] And, interestingly, adding rosemary extract to ground beef can reduce the formation of cancer-causing agents that may develop while cooking![32] Make sure to take some rosemary extract to your next barbecue!

IMPROVES HAIR

Historically, rosemary has been used to treat a variety of hair problems from hair loss to dandruff, making hair thicker and shinier, treating head lice, and even preventing graying of hair. When applied to the scalp, rosemary essential oil can help stimulate hair growth, and a 2015 study compared the effectiveness of rosemary oil to 2 percent minoxidil, otherwise known as Rogaine. The results showed that rosemary oil was as effective as Rogaine, and the patients in the rosemary group also experienced far fewer side effects compared to the minoxidil group. Both treatments seemed to produce significantly increased hair counts after six months of use. However, there is a big caveat. Rogaine users often use 5 percent minoxidil, rather than the 2 percent solution used in the study, thus skewing the results.[33] However, it's good to know that rosemary has some effect on preventing hair loss.

A different study looked at rosemary extract for the treatment of hair loss from testosterone use. The study was conducted on mice that were injected with hormones to induce varying degrees of baldness. The results were varying and found that rosemary could be promising for hair growth.[34]

More research looked into the effects of essential oils on baldness, specifically alopecia, a condition which leads to partial or complete absence of hair leading to baldness. The researchers looked into a mixture of essential oils, which included thyme, rosemary, lavender, and cedarwood. The mixture was massaged onto the scalps daily for seven months. They concluded that essential oils are a "safe and effective treatment for alopecia."[35] While not a blockbuster conclusion, this is good enough reason to go out and buy yourself some essential oils for a nice scalp rub.

STRESS

Who doesn't need a daily dose of stress-lowering goodness? Used in aromatherapy combined with other oils, rosemary can lower cortisol levels, thereby lowering anxiety. If you're having a stressful day, take a few drops and place in the palms of your hands. Rub the oil between your hands and take a few deep breaths in of the essential oil aroma.

Possible Side Effects, Contraindications, and Drug Interactions

Though generally considered safe, there have been occasional reports of allergic reactions to rosemary. Consuming excessively large amounts of rosemary leaves can cause serious side effects, including spasms, vomiting, pulmonary edema, and even coma. Pregnant and nursing women should not take rosemary as a supplement, but it is safe for them to eat as a spice in foods.

People with high blood pressure, ulcers, Crohn's disease, or ulcerative colitis should not take rosemary. Rosemary oil can be toxic if taken orally.

Rosemary may affect the blood's ability to clot, and could interfere with those who are on blood thinning drugs such as Warfarin and Clopidogrel. Rosemary may also interfere with the action of ACE inhibitors taken for blood pressure. If you are diabetic and are taking drugs to help control your diabetes, use precaution when consuming rosemary, as it may alter blood sugar levels and interfere with those drugs.

Rosemary Care Guide

Rosemary can be a tricky herb to grow indoors. The key to its survival is abundant sunlight and efficient watering practices. I've had many rosemary plants die in my hands, and it's not a fun road to discovery.

Rosemary is native to the Mediterranean, where there is plentiful sun, well-drained soil, and a lot of heat, along with moisture from the ocean air. Thus, it's no wonder that rosemary loves the sun but also needs enough moisture to keep it thriving. It's also important to note that growing rosemary outdoors in a garden is a completely different practice than growing it in containers. Below are instructions for container rosemary gardening.

Lighting: Rosemary needs full sun, indoors or outdoors. Make sure that if you are growing lavender indoors you have plenty of bright natural light.

Water: When inside a container, rosemary will need to be watered just enough. Yes, this is not a greatly detailed explanation, but here's the thing. Too much water is bad because it can lead to root rot, but too little water can also spell death. Make sure to water the soil at least every two weeks, but also make sure to check that the soil is dry first. And because rosemary likes to absorb water from the air (remember its ocean origins) make sure to place rocks or pebbles on the drainage pan for a more moist environment, and sit the pot on top of the rocks.

It's important to remember that indoor air is drier than outside. Rosemary enjoys moist foliage, and it would be good to take a spray bottle with water and mist the foliage about once or twice per week.

Soil: Known as an "upside down" plant, rosemary enjoys dry roots but moist foliage, and will want to absorb moisture from its leaves. When growing this plant in a container, you will need to have drainage holes and well-draining soil. Use cactus soil mix or something similar.

Remedies

Rosemary Oil

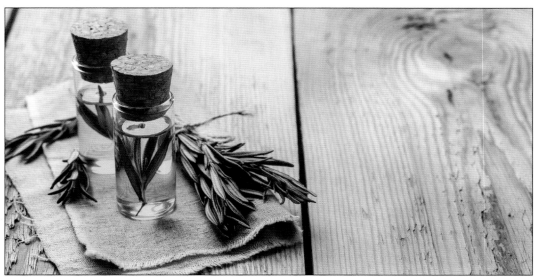

Rosemary oil is a great way to get all the important essences out of your rosemary plant for the ultimate healing benefits. Use as a moisturizer for your skin, a massage oil, or rub it into your scalp to stimulate hair growth.

Ingredients:

- Fresh rosemary
- Mason jars
- Olive oil or jojoba oil
- 1-ounce glass bottles with droppers

Instructions:

1. Pick your fresh rosemary, wash it, and let it completely dry. Cut enough to fill up a mason jar. Cutting and crushing the rosemary will bring out the aroma and various oils in the herb.
2. Fill up your mason jar with your freshly cut and clean rosemary.
3. Fill your jar with your oil of choice, completely covering the plant. I like to use olive oil or jojoba.
4. Place your jar on a windowsill that gets plenty of sun, for about a month.
5. After a month, strain your oil into a clean jar and throw away any pieces of the plant that have been separated during straining.
6. Fill your 1-ounce bottles with your rosemary oil and label the bottles!

If you keep your bottle closed tightly and out of direct sun, the oil should last you for up to six months.

Rosemary Shampoo

Using the rosemary oil recipe above, you can quickly make your own hair stimulating shampoo that not only smells great, but helps rejuvenate your follicly challenged scalp.

Ingredients:

- ¼ cup distilled water
- 2 tablespoons dried rosemary
- shampoo bottles
- ¼ cup liquid castile soap
- 1 teaspoon vegetable glycerin
- ½ teaspoon jojoba oil
- 7 drops rosemary oil
- 5 drops peppermint oil

Instructions:

1. Boil the distilled water in a pot and remove from heat. Steep 2 tablespoons of dried rosemary for twenty minutes.
2. After twenty minutes, strain the rosemary tea, let it cool down completely, and pour it into a shampoo bottle.
3. Using a funnel, pour the liquid castile soap into the bottle, followed by the vegetable glycerin, jojoba oil, and rosemary and peppermint oils.
4. Close the bottle and shake well to combine.
5. Your homemade rosemary shampoo is done, simple as that. Store your shampoo in a cool, dry place, preferably the refrigerator, and use within a month. Shake well before each use.

Rosemary Digestive Tea

A great way to use your homegrown rosemary is to make your own tea! Additionally, this is the perfect way to aid your digestion before and after meals.

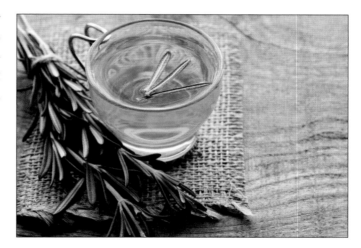

Ingredients:

- 1–2 fresh sprigs of rosemary, or 1–1½ teaspoons of dried rosemary
- 2 cups boiling water
- Honey (optional)

Instructions:

Break up your rosemary into small pieces and boil them in a pan with water and honey. Reduce the heat when it is fully at a boil, and let sit for five minutes. After the time is up, strain out the water from the mixture.

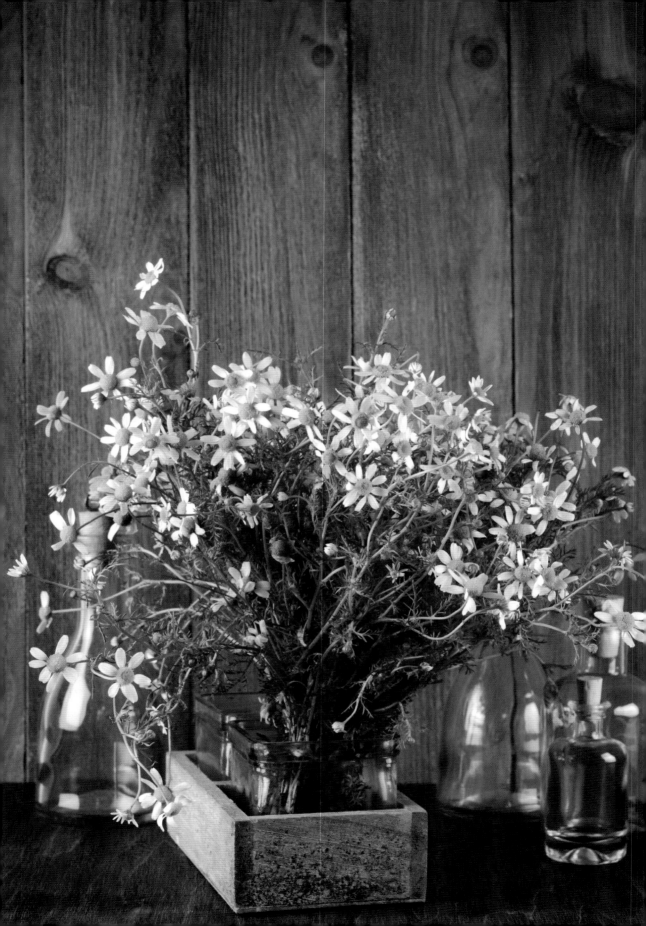

Chapter Six: Chamomile

Matricaria chamomilla

Chamomile is a wonderful and versatile herb, sweet tasting and lacking the bitterness of many other herbal remedies. It has been a healing medicinal for thousands of years, a trusted and very valued herbal remedy. The word *chamomile* is derived from French, Latin, and Greek, meaning "earth apple," "on the ground," and, simply, "apple."

A member of the Asteraceae/ Compositae family, chamomile has two widely known and common varieties, German chamomile and Roman chamomile. And while these two varieties come from difference species, the word *chamomile* actually refers to a range of different daisy-like plants.

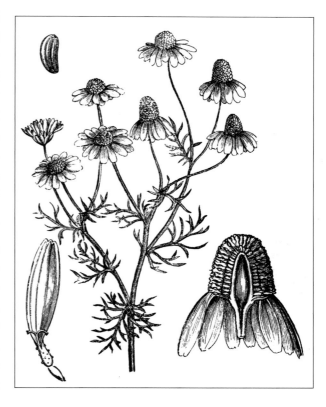

Native to Europe and northern Africa, chamomile was used throughout the ancient world, including ancient Rome, Greece, and Egypt. Chamomile is cultivated worldwide today and has a wide variety of applications. Used as a form of medicine for at least five thousand years, it's been traditionally used for insomnia, anxiety, acne, digestive disorders, chest colds, bruises, burns, sciatica, rheumatic pain, hemorrhoids, sore throats, and more.

Ancient hieroglyphic records show that chamomile was used cosmetically for at least two thousand years, and Greek physicians prepared chamomile as a way to treat fevers and women's health. In fact, chamomile was widely used for its ability to ease menstrual cramps and pain in childbirth. And while you may have sipped on chamomile tea throughout your life, little did you know it does way more than just calm the nerves and help you sleep.

Health Benefits

ANTI-INFLAMMATORY PROPERTIES

If you suffer from pain or any type of inflammation, chamomile has the answer you've been looking for. Sometimes called the "herbal aspirin," chamomile has specific anti-inflammatory properties, which can help treat pain. This herb is able to treat the root of the problem, addressing the symptom of pain with its actual cause: inflammation. This natural painkiller can help with conditions such as arthritis, back pain, fevers, and more.

Chamomile essential oil is often added to skincare products due to its ability to treat skin irritations, facial swelling, toothaches, and more. Its various volatile oils such as alpha-bisabolol, alpha-bisabolol oxides A and B, and matricin, are what make chamomile so effective. A review of the plant published in *Molecular Medicine Reports* in 2010 found that chamomile flavonoids and chamomile essential oils are able to "penetrate below the skin surface into the deeper skin layers." This is important as it can work as a topical anti-inflammatory more successfully than other oils or herbs.

FIGHTS CANCER

Research has shown that chamomile helps stop cancerous tumor growth. This may be due to an antioxidant called apigenin, which has been found to help stop various cancers, including skin, prostate, breast, and ovarian. A study from Ohio State University found that apigenin can prevent breast cancer cells from reproducing and spreading, basically normalizing cancer cells.[36]

A different study in the *Journal of Agriculture and Food Chemistry* found that extracts from chamomile cause apoptosis, or cell death, in cancer cells, which inhibits their growth. However, in normal cells, chamomile does not promote apoptosis, making it an amazing remedy that is able to recognize and seek out cancer.[37] Chamomile is like a missile, tracking and categorically killing the bad guys.

PROMOTES CARDIOVASCULAR HEALTH

It's been shown that foods and herbs which contain flavonoids may be useful in treating cardiovascular conditions. One study followed 805 elderly men between the ages of sixty-five and eighty-four and found that the men who had higher intakes of flavonoid-rich foods and herbs had a lower mortality rate from coronary heart disease.[38]

Promotes Gastrointestinal Health

It may come as no surprise that chamomile has benefits for the gastrointestinal system. Many of us have been told to snuggle up with a cup of chamomile tea when we are feeling bloated or have an upset stomach. Traditionally it's been used to help get rid of gas, soothe stomach pain, and alleviate any type of stomach irritation. And there's research to back this up. Chamomile has been found to shorten the course of diarrhea in children and relieve the symptoms as well. It's also been shown to be helpful in cases of colic. Chamomile tea prepared with licorice, fennel, balm mint, and vervain was found useful to treat colic in 57 percent of infants, compared to 26 percent of infants treated with placebo[39]. It's also been found to be helpful in the treatment of irritable bowel syndrome in adults.

Alleviates Eczema

With its amazing anti-inflammatory properties and the ability to enter deeper layers of the skin, chamomile is the ultimate remedy for skin conditions, especially eczema. Topical applications of chamomile have been found to be about 60 percent as effective as hydrocortisone cream, but without all the side effects. Roman chamomile has been specifically shown to reduce discomfort related to eczema when applied as a cream containing chamomile extract.

Sleep Aid

Go to the grocery store and pick up any kind of sleep-promoting tea and you're bound to find chamomile in it. It's almost ubiquitous when it comes to herbal sleep aids, and for good reason: it works. Chamomile has long been used as a mild tranquilizer and sleep inducer. Some studies show chamomile to be a central nervous system depressant and some extracts have been shown to act similarly to benzodiazepine-like hypnotic activity.

Reduces Anxiety

When it comes to reducing anxiety and living a calmer, more relaxed life, chamomile might be one solution. In 2009, the University of Pennsylvania conducted a randomized, double-blind, placebo-controlled trial to test the effects chamomile has on general anxiety. While the study was small, it brought back interesting results. Fifty-nine participants over eight weeks were given either chamomile capsules with 220 mg of pharmaceutical-grade German chamomile or a placebo pill containing lactose. Chamomile compared favorably with placebo, and its results were statistically significant.[40]

Possible Side Effects, Contraindications, and Drug Interactions

Chamomile is generally considered safe. However, in some circumstances, chamomile may make asthma worse. Pregnant women should also avoid using chamomile.

Chamomile may cause drowsiness, so do not operate a car or heavy machinery after taking chamomile.

Chamomile may also increase the risk of bleeding. If you currently take blood-thinning medications such as Warfarin, Clopidogrel, and aspirin, please remain cautious.

Because of chamomile's sedative abilities, you should be cautious when taking antiseizure drugs, barbiturates, benzodiazepines, and sleeping pills.

Chamomile may slightly lower blood pressure, so if you currently take blood pressure medications be cautious, as it could make your blood pressure drop too low.

Chamomile also may naturally lower blood sugar, so be careful if you are taking a drug to manage diabetes.

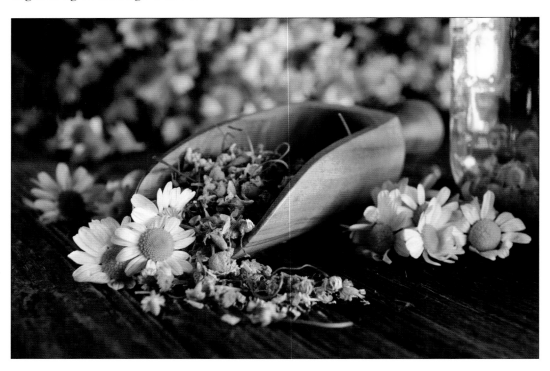

Chamomile Care Guide

Growing chamomile indoors is an easy way to have a year-round supply of this amazing herbal remedy, and it's not that hard! Great news—chamomile can be grown and planted in the winter, as it only requires around four hours of sunlight per day. The plant will be fine as long as it is sitting in a southward-facing window. You'll be able to harvest your flowers after around sixty to ninety days. This herb is hardy and won't need a lot of extra care, so don't worry about fancy potting soils or fertilizers; your chamomile will be hardy and strong.

Light: Chamomile needs around four hours of light per day. Make sure the pot is sitting in a southward-facing window.

Water: You should only water your chamomile around once per week. The soil should be kept moist, but not too wet.

Remedies

Sleepy Time Chamomile Tincture

This easy-to-make chamomile tincture is a safe and simple way to help your body relax and fall asleep naturally. A dose right before bedtime will relax the mind and body and help you drift off smoothly. Chamomile tinctures can be found widely online or in stores, but if you're looking for a cheaper and homemade option, this is a wonderful recipe. For adults, take up to one teaspoon, one to three times a day or as needed.

Ingredients:

- ½ cup dried chamomile flowers
- Glass jar with airtight lid, quart size
- 1¾ cups boiling water
- 1¾ cups vodka
- cheesecloth
- Tincture vial with droppers

Directions:

1. Place your dried chamomile flowers in your clean and sterile glass jar.
2. Pour boiling water over the flowers, making sure you just cover them.

3. Fill the rest of the jar with the vodka of your choice. Cover the jar with an airtight lid.
4. Store the jar in a cool and dark place for four to six weeks. I like placing the jars in my kitchen cabinets.
5. After four to six weeks, take your jar and strain the liquid out into a cheesecloth or strainer. Once the liquid is separated out from the flowers, you have your tincture. Place the liquid in a tincture vial with dropper.

DIY Chamomile Flower Tea for Anxiety and Stress

Drinking three cups of chamomile tea per day can help you relieve some anxiety and stress, while also reducing your inflammation and pain! This one-stop shop of herbal goodness is an easy way to incorporate herbal medicine, and it tastes good! Chamomile is unique in its sweet and fruity taste. Using an infuser pot to brew your tea is an easy way to make fresh tea using loose leaves. If you don't have an infuser teapot, find a strainer or cheesecloth in order to make a makeshift tea bag.

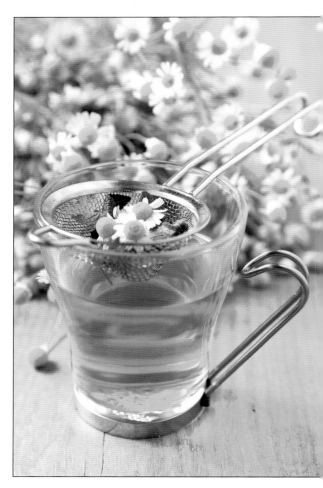

Ingredients:

- 3–4 tablespoons fresh chamomile flowers
- 1 sprig fresh mint
- 8 ounces boiling water

Instructions:

1. Harvest your chamomile flowers the same day you plan to use them for tea. Pop the heads of the flowers off the stems, and mix together with fresh mint sprig.
2. Boil your 8 ounces of water and place it in your teapot with the herbs, or over the cheesecloth. Steep your flowers and mint in the water for five minutes.

DIY Chamomile Skin Toner

Chamomile flowers combined with an assortment of essential oils will provide a gentle and effective toner for your skin. Help alleviate rashes, redness, inflammation, and itchiness with this amazing concoction.

Ingredients:

- 1 cup water
- 3 tablespoons dried chamomile flowers
- ¼ cup witch hazel
- 5 drops sweet orange essential oil
- 2 drops peppermint essential oil

Instructions:

1. Boil the water and pour over your dried chamomile flowers. Steep for ten minutes and strain off the flowers. Cool the tea to room temperature.
2. Combine the cool and concentrated chamomile tea with the witch hazel and essential oils. Transfer the mixture into a glass bottle for storage.
3. Apply the toner to your face after washing and rinsing by using a cotton ball. Apply liberally while avoiding contact with the eyes.
4. Allow your face to air dry.

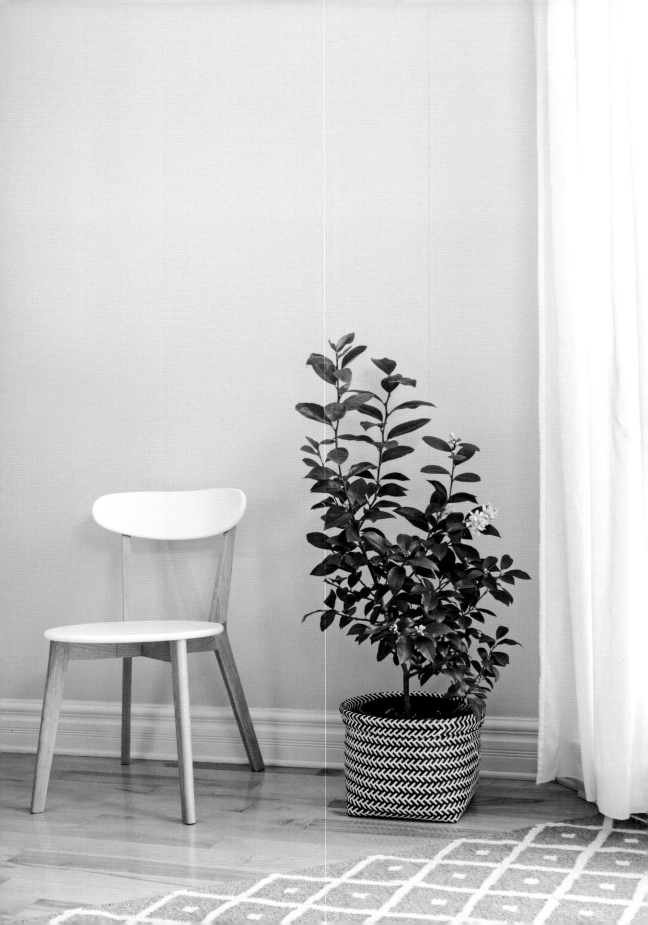

Chapter Seven: Lemon Tree

Citrus limon

Lemons often bring forth images of sunshine and warm weather, but lemon trees are wonderful house-plants that thrive through all seasons—even winter. When put in the correct container, these plants will do just fine in the winter while they wait out the cold. Lemons are also more than just a garnish for your gin and tonic; they have wonderful healing capabilities and were consumed on ships to prevent the all-too-common ailment among sailors—scurvy. Currently, research has shown lemons lower the risk of stroke, fight formation of free radicals that are known to cause

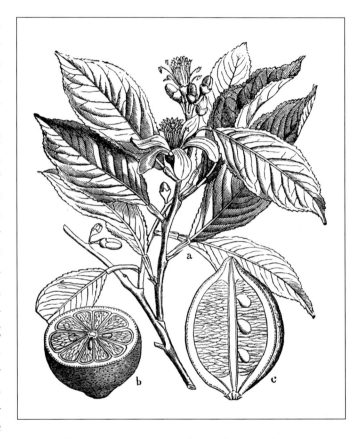

cancer, help maintain a healthy complexion, prevent asthma, boost the immune system, and more.

While lemons and limes are considered staples in your homemade bar, they've been used for healing since the ancient Egyptians and Syrians. People have been cultivating citrus for over four thousand years, and while we associate lemons with limoncello in the Mediterranean, the origins are actually native to India and China, where it's found growing wild and used as an antiseptic and antirheumatic. We can credit the spread of lemons and our love of lemon sorbet to Arab traders who first brought these delicious fruits to Sicily around 200 AD.

Lemons provide 187 percent of the recommended daily value of vitamin C, plus great amounts of potassium, calcium, folate, B6, magnesium, and copper. Lemons also have flavonoid glycosides called esperetin and naringenin, which are known to kill free radicals in the body, which have been linked to cholesterol buildup, atherosclerosis, and heart disease. Their high levels of citric acid, which is converted to citrate in the body, can also get converted into precursors for something called acetylcholine, which is important for REM sleep, learning, and memory.

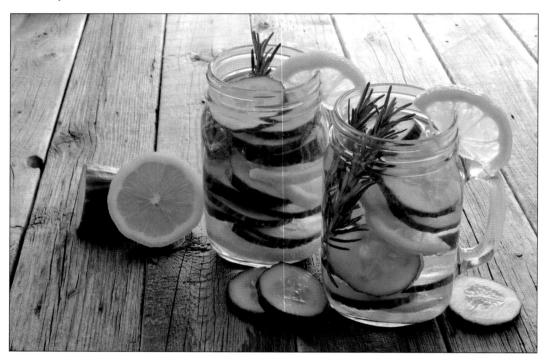

Health Benefits

BOOSTS IMMUNITY

A major benefit of consuming a food high in vitamin C is its ability to regulate the immune system and help wage attacks against those nasty bugs that cause colds and flu. If you want to boost your immunity and prepare yourself for cold and flu season, start ingesting a lot of lemon!

ANTI-INFLAMMATORY PROPERTIES

Like most plants, lemons are known to be anti-inflammatories. A compound called beta-cryptoxanthin, found in lemons, has been shown to be a factor in reducing inflammatory diseases such as rheumatoid arthritis.

REDUCE YOUR RISK OF KIDNEY STONES

As a member of the citrus family, lemons are high in citric acid. Actually, out of all the citrus fruits, lemons have the highest concentration of citric acid, containing around 8 percent of the dry weight of a lemon. It's been shown that citric acid may be beneficial in slowing the formation of kidney stones and may help stop these crystals from turning into bigger ones. Essentially, the more citric acid you have in your urine the more protected you are from forming these painful problems.

LOWERED RISK OF STROKE

Probably the most surprising benefit of lemons is their potential ability to lower the risk of stroke in women. According to the American Heart Association, those who eat higher amounts of citrus, including lemon, have a lower risk of ischemic stroke than those who consumed the least. The study looked at over 69,622 women over a fourteen-year time period. This benefit may be from lemon's high levels of vitamin C, which is associated with lower levels of stroke due to its protection on various levels, including improving blood vessel function and acting as an anti-inflammatory.[41]

Possible Side Effects, Contraindications, and Drug Interactions

Lemons are generally very safe, and no amount of lemon sorbet will wreak very much havoc. However, as with anything, you should take precautions. In larger amounts, lemon juice may cause GERD and ulcers, which may be triggered by acidic foods.

Lemon juice can cause tooth enamel to decay, leading to stained teeth, loss of dental tissue, and, in some cases, cavities.

Those who are currently taking medications should also check with their doctor for any interactions.

Lemon Tree Care Guide

You might believe it's impossible to have a lemon tree if you're stuck in the great white north, but in reality, we can all have thriving lemon trees in our homes. Yes, they may be cold sensitive, but that's no reason to avoid growing these beautiful reminders of warmer weather and thawed-out limbs. These trees grow great in containers as long as you supply a pot that's big enough to provide adequate drainage and room for their growth. You can expect your lemon tree to grow from around three to five feet tall.

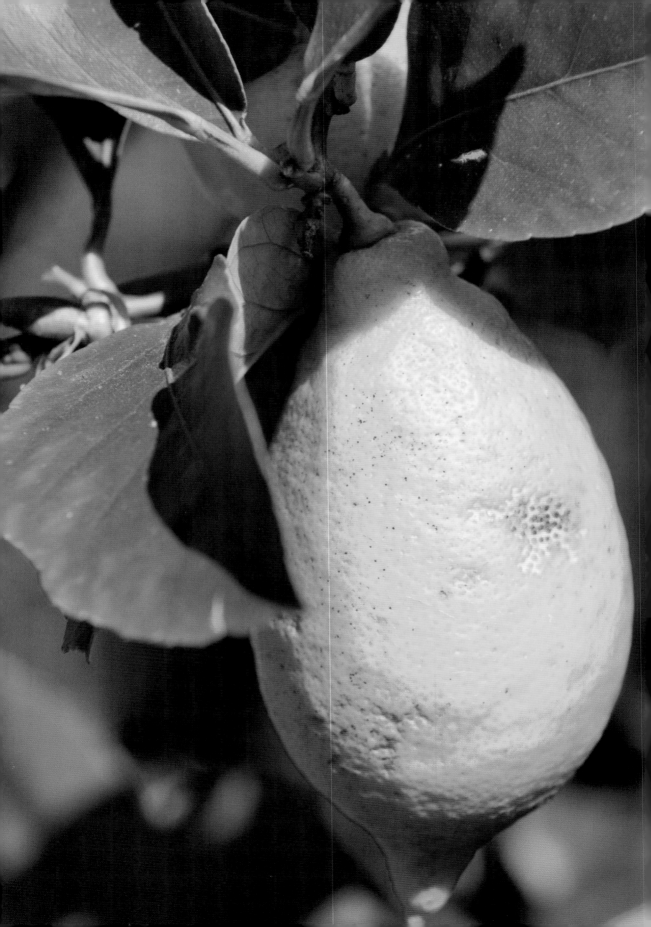

Lighting: Your lemon tree will need a lot of light. Make sure you place them near a southward-facing window, and if you live in a climate with short days in the winter, you might want to purchase a fluorescent grow light for the season.

Water: Make sure to keep the soil evenly moist. Don't let it get too dry, and of course, never overwater. With container citrus trees, make sure to water as soon as the soil dries out or if it is only slightly damp, and never let your lemon tree dry out for more than one day.

Temperature: Lemon trees will thrive the best in temperatures around 70°F during the day and 55°F at night.

Soil: Lemon trees need well-draining soil that is slightly acidic. Keep the soil moist and fertilize during the growing season.

Summer Months: During the warmer months, lemon trees can be placed outside, which will be beneficial to helping them grow their fruit. Placing them outside will also increase their visibility to bees, allowing them to be pollinated.

Recipes and Remedies

Lemon Water

If you're looking for the least amount of work for the highest reward, lemon water just might be your next favorite thing. Lemon water is a wonderful way to get your daily dose of vitamin C while also sneaking in a serving of magnesium, copper, and potassium.

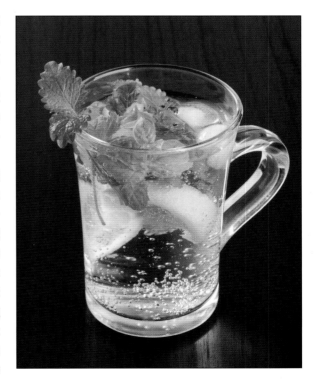

Lemon water makes drinking water more enticing, giving it a refreshing twist on the most boring drink in the books. Drinking a glass of fresh lemon water in the morning will help aid in digestion and tell your liver to produce more bile, which keeps foods moving through your gastrointestinal tract smoothly. Lemon water can also help provide steady insulin levels and increased absorption of nutrients. The antioxidants in this simple drink will fight damage caused by free radicals and keep you looking fresh and your skin looking young. A study published in the *American Journal of Clinical Nutrition* found that consuming vitamin C on a regular basis keeps your skin looking younger with fewer wrinkles.[42]

Not to mention, if you're worried about getting kidney stones, or have a history of them, drink lemon water every day to help prevent and fight those dreadful stones! Doctors are now calling it "lemonade therapy"!

Ingredients:

- 1 lemon
- 24 ounces warm water
- 5 mint leaves (optional)

Instructions:

1. Zest your lemon and store it in the freezer for future recipes.
2. Cut the lemon in half and squeeze the whole lemon into your water.
3. Take your mint leaves and put them in the water. To get the most taste, muddle the leaves at the bottom to break up the essential oils of the mint.
4. Drink!

Chest Congestion and Sinus Remedy

If you're already sick and suffering, it's important to take care of yourself and make sure to ingest the healthiest foods out there. This very simple remedy will help soothe your throat, boost your immune system, and decrease your mucus buildup.

Ingredients:

- 1 mug of hot water
- 2 tablespoons lemon juice
- 2 teaspoons apple cider vinegar
- 1 teaspoon honey

Instructions:

Heat the water to boiling and place in a mug. Mix the lemon juice, apple cider vinegar, and honey into the hot water. This easy and refreshing drink will help with congestion, mucus, and phlegm and will boost your immune system and soothe your throat. Drink a few times a day when sick.

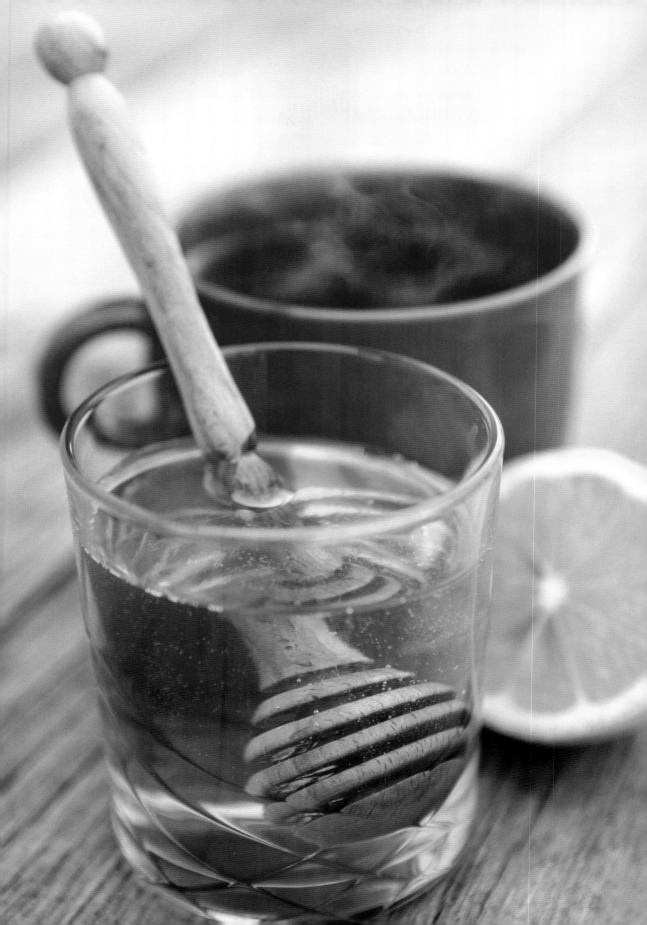

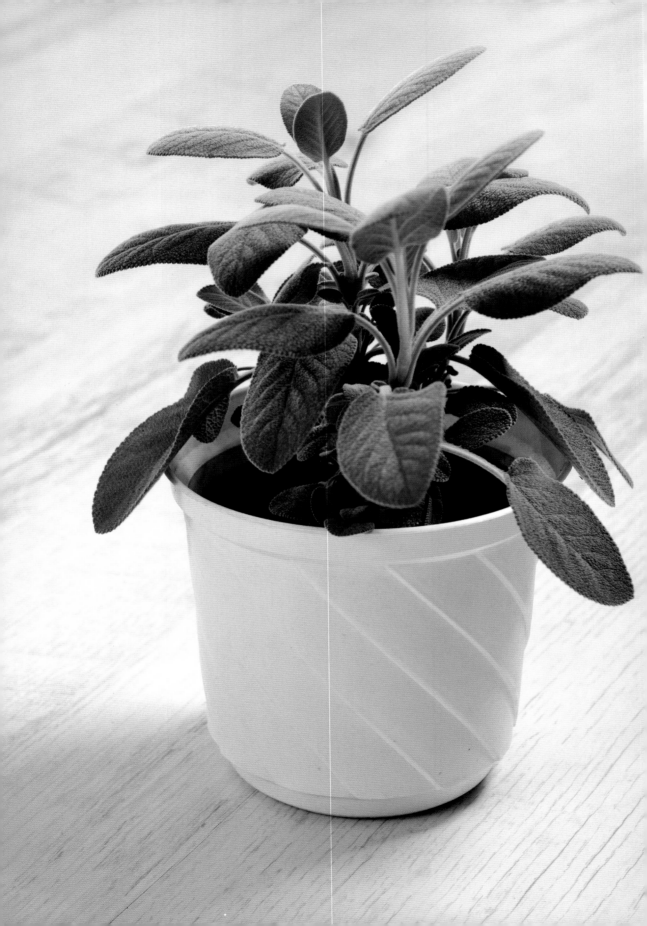

Chapter Eight: Sage

Salvia officinalis

Sage is often used by healers and homeowners as a way to cleanse and heal spaces and to get rid of that weird smell in the kitchen. Sage is easily grown indoors, assuming there is plenty of sunlight around, and its health benefits abound. A relative of rosemary, the botanical name comes from the Latin word *salvere*, meaning "to be saved."

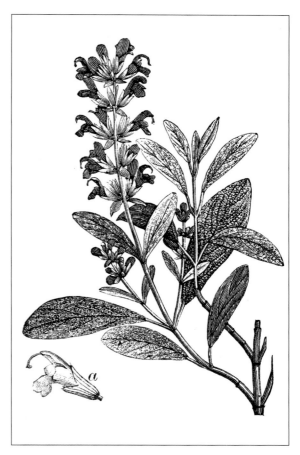

Used throughout the centuries, this herb has been beloved by the Romans, Charlemagne in France, the ancient Egyptians, the ancient Greeks, and the ancient Chinese. Should I forget an ancient culture that loved sage dearly, I truly apologize, but this plant is just too darn popular. Not to mention, sage also has a wide range of uses, from aiding digestion to cleaning ulcers and wounds; stopping bleeding; treating sprains or a hoarse voice; regulating women's menstrual cycles; improving memory; alleviating sore throats, coughs, and the common cold; and more.

Throughout the ages, sage has been considered somewhat of a panacea, being of utmost value in the herbal medicine cabinets throughout history's most important cultures and healers. Today, sage is often used for muscle aches, rheumatism, aromatherapy, increasing memory, mental clarity, and treating cognitive decline. Its tea is known as "thinker's tea" and even eases depression. To get the most out of the medicinally diverse plant, many ingest it by eating, drinking (as a tea), or making it into a tincture.

The Art of Burning Sage

The art and ritual of burning herbs is a tradition used in many cultures throughout millennia. From burning frankincense in the Bible to the incredibly popular nag champa incense in every Phish-loving college dorm, almost all cultures have a tradition of cleansing spaces, or people, with burning or smudging herbs. The most popular herb is sage, from the Native American tradition. As with all ancient and cultural traditions, it's important to practice smudging with respect. If you're wary of or cynical about this ancient practice, read on to learn more about sage's healing properties.

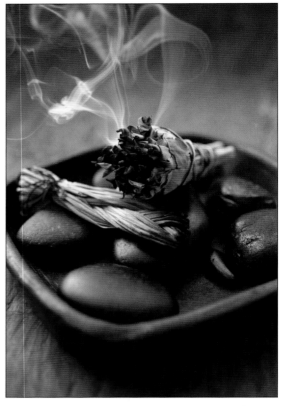

The ritual of smudging your spaces is said to be an energetic cleansing and spiritual practice that allows for meditation and helps connect you to the spiritual world. For those who don't resonate with this idea, just stay with me. Native Americans have used dried white sage to reset and purify spaces for over two thousand years, believing that it absorbs anger, conflict, or bad energy. You can think of smudging as a way to clean, similar to washing your hands or taking a shower. And smudging isn't just good for the soul; it's been proven to purify the air from harmful germs and bacteria.

Recent research has shown that the art of smudging is more than just a superstitious practice, but a proven germ killer with clinical benefits. A 2006 review titled "Medicinal Smokes" from the *Journal of Ethnopharmacology* looked at over fifty countries that used single- and multi-ingredient herbal remedies that were administered with smoke and found that these cultures used this technique for pulmonary, neurological, and dermatological needs. They realized that this type of "passive smoke" was also commonly used as an air purifier.

The researchers found that inhaling smoke was an advantageous way to ingest medicine, as it provides rapid delivery to the brain, making it a particularly efficient way for medicine to be absorbed by the body.[43] Realizing that there was more to smudging than previously recognized, the researchers published another paper eleven months later titled "Medicinal Smoke Reduces Airborne Bacteria," produced in the same journal. What the researchers found was quite impressive. They found that burning medicinal herbs can clear the air of bacteria by 94 percent in one hour, with the room being decontaminated in twenty-four hours. Even more, one month later, the room still had no trace of seven other pathogenic bacteria.[44]

This is quite impressive, especially since many of us live in cities which contain over 1,800 different types of airborne bacteria, many of which are pathogenic and can be passed along quite easily. So the next time you come down with something contagious, be kind and smudge your space! If you want your loved one stopping by with chicken noodle soup, you can at least clear the air of your gross, sickly air particles.

Health Benefits

The many health properties of sage don't just come in the form of burning, but also from ingesting. Sage has anti-inflammatory and antiseptic properties; it also contains a wide array of volatile oils and can be used medicinally for a variety of ailments including muscle aches, rheumatism, depression, asthma, and even atherosclerosis. Sage also includes many vitamins and minerals, including vitamin K, vitamin A, folate, magnesium, manganese, calcium, folic acid, riboflavin, copper, vitamin C, and vitamin E.

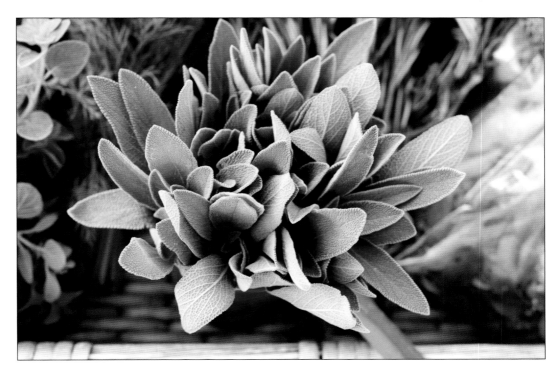

IMPROVES MEMORY

One small study found sage to be a useful treatment in enhancing memory and cognition. This placebo-controlled, double-blind study showed significant improvement in word and cognitive recall immediately following and several hours after ingestion of sage compared to the placebo group. Those who were given the sage oil tablets were found to be significantly better at word recall than those who weren't.[45] Spanish sage has been shown to be effective in enhancing the speed of memory and improving mood.

Other studies have shown sage to be effective in treating memory disorders and cognitive decline. Traditional Chinese medicine uses Chinese sage as a restorative of lost and declining mental function, such as Alzheimer's disease. Sage essential oil has been found to inhibit the enzyme acetyl cholinesterase by 46 percent. This enzyme is known to inactivate acetylcholine, which leads to Alzheimer's.

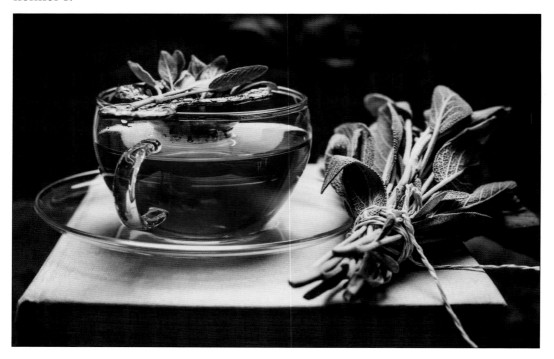

ANTI-INFLAMMATORY PROPERTIES

More recently, research has shown[46] that two plant-derived compounds from sage known as diterpenoids are potent anti-inflammatories and could help treat pain. The two compounds, known as carnosol and carnosic acid, are known to interfere with the pathways related to pain and inflammation in the body. This breakthrough could mean that sage is a safer and nonaddictive approach to treating pain than most mainstream methods.

COMBATS DIABETES

Cultures throughout the world have used sage to combat diabetes, and there's research to corroborate these methods. Studies on animals have shown many glucose-lowering effects. In one study, drinking sage tea twice a day showed an improved lipid profile without any side effects.[47] And one study showed that sage extract had a hypoglycemic effect in diabetic animals, but more research is needed.[48]

EASES SYMPTOMS OF MENOPAUSE

For those experiencing hot flashes, you may want to add sage to your toolbox of aids. A study conducted in Switzerland found that a preparation of fresh sage reduced the number of hot flashes by 50 percent in four weeks and 64 percent in eight weeks in participants who experienced at least five hot flashes daily.[49]

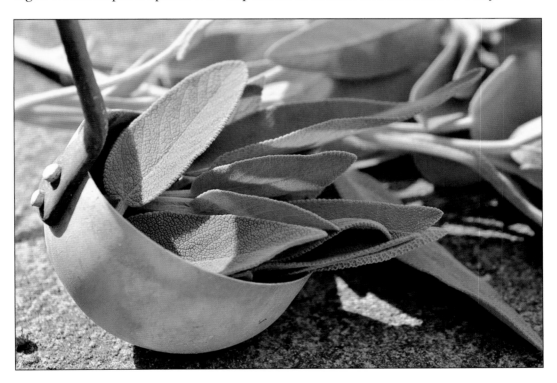

Possible Side Effects, Contraindications, and Drug Interactions

Generally recognized as safe by the Food and Drug Administration, sage is commonly found as a spice for food or used in seasonings. Some species of sage, however, contain a compound called thujone, which can affect the nervous system. Large amounts of ingestion or extended use can lead to vomiting, vertigo, restlessness, tremors, increased heart rate, and even kidney damage. Ingesting sage essential oil may be toxic.

Some possible drug interactions to be aware of include diabetic drugs, due to sage's ability to lower blood sugar. Antiseizure medications and sedative medications could also be interactive, as sage may cause drowsiness and sleepiness. If you are currently taking sedative medications, including clonazepam, lorazepam, phenobarbital, zolpidem, and others, please remain cautious.

Sage Care Guide

If you want the most economical way to enjoy and use sage, grow it yourself. It's an easy plant to keep healthy due to the herb's hardy nature and drought-tolerant qualities. It also grows well in a wide range of temperatures and climates, and has a long growing season. You'll be harvesting this herb well into the fall, and best of all, sage will do great in containers! Sage is also special because it's one of the few herbs whose flavor intensifies as the leaves grow larger.

Lighting: Sage needs lots of light, so make sure it's placed in a part of the house with full sun.

Water: This hardy and drought-tolerant plant will do best if you let the soil dry in between watering. Never let it sit in soggy soil (but do water when the soil gets fully dry) and you'll do just fine.

Temperature: Sage will do well indoors as long as it's kept away from cold drafts.

Soil: Make sure your sage lives in well-draining soil that's sandy or loamy.

Recipes and Remedies

Sage Smudge Stick

Making your own sage smudge sticks is a fun and easy way to use your supply of herbs, and they don't have to be relegated to your sage. This is a fun way to mix and match different herbs that you are growing, from lavender to rose petals to mugwort. For this recipe, the main herb we'll use is sage (obviously), but feel free to sprinkle in other herbs with aromas you find delicious and enticing.

However, when it comes to burning sage, you should only burn white sage. Common sage can be unsafe to burn, and other seemingly benign culinary herbs can set off allergic or asthmatic reactions when burned. When it comes to other herbs, make sure you test them out, burning a small dose outdoors to make sure their smell isn't overwhelming and noxious. Some people have negative reactions to different herbs; it's a true trial-and-error game.

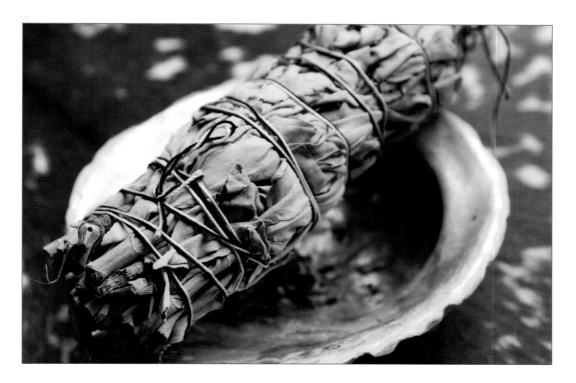

Some common herbs that would make great smudge sticks include white sage, thyme, yarrow, juniper, pine, lavender, lemon balm, mint, bee balm, catnip, mugwort, cedar, sweetgrass, and sagebrush.

Ingredients:

- Herb(s) of your choice
- 100 percent natural string or twine (Remember, this will burn too. Make sure it's safe.)

Instructions:

1. Harvest and gather your herbs on the same day you want to create a smudge stick (remember that it will need to dry for a few weeks after you make it and before you use it). Make sure your herbs aren't moist, or else there is a good chance of growing mold on the inside of the bundle.
2. Place the stems of the herbs together, making sure those with similar lengths are clipped alongside one another. Try to make your bundle on the thicker side, around 1½ to 2 inches wide, as the leaves will shrink and become smaller as time goes on.
3. Wrap the string around the stems of the herbs and secure with a knot. Then wrap around again and tie another knot to make sure it's secure.

4. Begin winding the string around the bundle spiraling up. Pull tightly as you go, and once you reach the top continue wrapping, crisscrossing down towards the base. Tie the loose end at the stem.

5. Hang your fresh smudge stick for up to three weeks for drying. After three weeks it's time to use your smudge sticks! There are many ways to use a sage stick, from "cleansing" your new home by waving the lit stick around every room of the house, to simply letting it sit in a fireproof dish once lit for an incense-type effect.

Sage Oil

Sage oil has a wide range of benefits and can help you with skin disorders, regulate your menstrual cycle, clean wounds, reduce inflammation, and more. In a study published in the *Brazilian Journal of Microbiology*, it was found that several oils have antimicrobial properties against vancomycin-resistant enterococci and *Escherichia coli* strains. However, out of all the tested oils, they found that thyme and sage essential oils showed the most significant results against these bacteria.[50]

Making sage oil will be useful in other DIY home remedies and will be a great base to have for a number of projects. Use it as a massage oil to help relax muscles, rub along the lower stomach to help reduce menstrual cramps, vaporize it for aromatherapy purposes, and more. Get creative with this amazing herb and use it for a variety of purposes.

Ingredients:

- 1 cup fresh sage
- Freezer bag
- Rubber mallet
- Glass jar with a wide mouth
- ½ cup olive oil
- Strainer
- Funnel
- Colored glass container

Instructions:

1. Harvest a cup of fresh sage and place it in a freezer bag. Seal the bag and pound it using a rubber mallet.

2. Put the crushed sage in a wide-mouth glass container and add half a cup of olive oil. Seal it and place the jar in a warm place where the sun will touch it. Leave it for forty-eight hours.

3. Strain the oil from the mixture and put it back into the jar. Discard the sage leaves.

4. If you want to create a more potent version of sage oil, repeat the first three steps.
5. When done, place the sage oil in a colored glass jar in order to slow the aging process. Place it in a cabinet or a refrigerator.

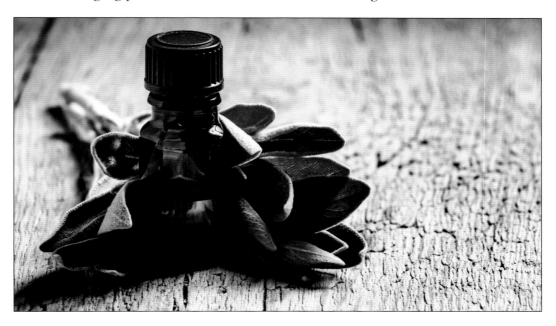

Sage Butter

If you want to taste the most delicious butter, one that becomes the central part of your meal and gets all the glory and attention, try sage butter. Incredibly simple to make and an excuse to eat more butter, this sage-filled recipe also uses a mix of other ingredients to make your mouth feel like it's having a party.

Ingredients:

- ½ cup fresh sage leaves
- 1 large shallot
- ½ cup butter, soft
- 1 teaspoon fresh lemon juice
- ¼ teaspoon freshly ground pepper

Instructions:

Put the sage and shallot in a food processor until all is chopped. Add the butter and the remaining ingredients; process until the mixture is blended thoroughly. When done, place the mixture in a small bowl and feel free to refrigerate to harden. Use on bread, crackers, chips, or anything that makes it easier to get this butter into your mouth.

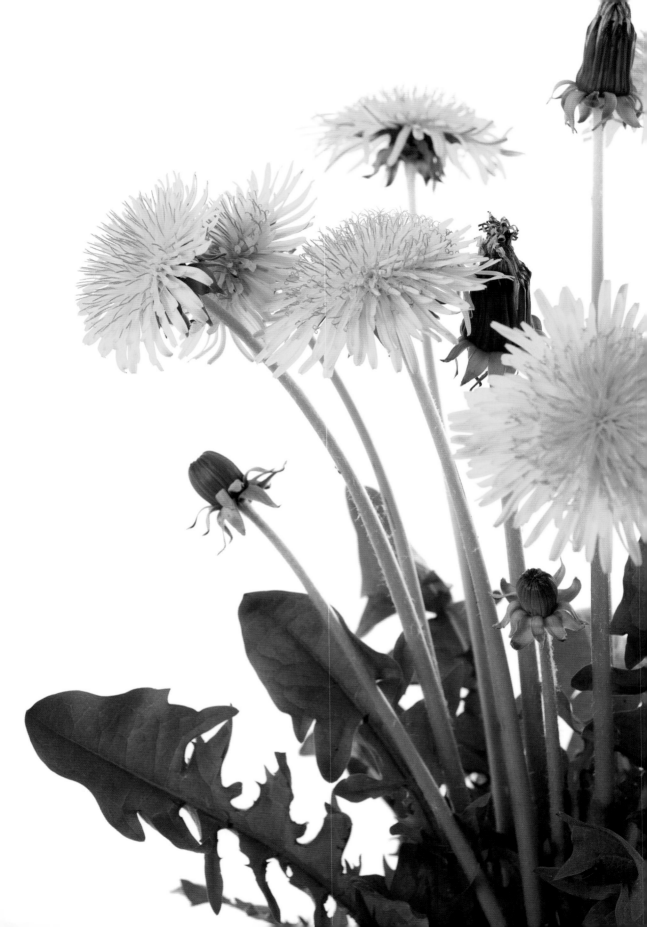

Chapter Nine: Dandelion

Taraxacum

Often thought of as a pesky weed, it's time to flip the script on this amazing plant. Dandelion is one of the most important plants in herbal medicine, used for a wide variety of ailments. Chinese medicine has been ingesting dandelion for over a thousand years, using it as a remedy for many ailments, including diabetes, cancer, bacterial infections, fevers, skin conditions, and more.

The Native Americans also loved dandelion for its ability to treat renal conditions, skin disorders, and even heartburn. European traditions used dandelion to treat diabetes, eye disorders, fevers, boils, and in Ayurveda they use dandelion for various liver disorders, such as jaundice, cirrhosis, and enlargement.

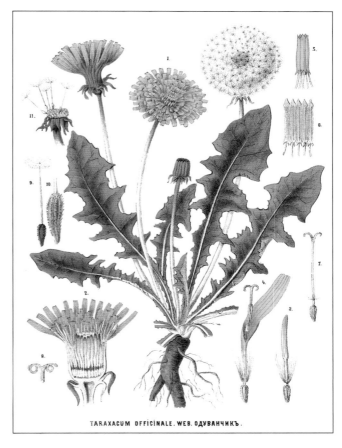

TARAXACUM OFFICINALE. WEB. ОДУВАНЧИКЪ.

The weed that takes over your lawn has been shown to be rich in vitamin C, fiber, potassium, calcium, iron, magnesium, zinc, B-complex vitamins, trace minerals, and phosphorus. And before you start weed whacking, you might want to keep dandelion around for your garden. Dandelions are actually beneficial weeds, as they bring nutrients to the top of the soil, which can help your shallow-rooted plants thrive. Dandelions also add extra minerals and nitrogen to the soil, not to mention that they attract pollinating insects.

Native to Eurasia, the common dandelion is part of the sunflower family. Dandelions have two major phases of life, with which we are all familiar: prebloom and postbloom. Prebloom dandelions are a poor man's beautiful bouquet, bright and sunny yellow flowers, known to every cheap date as free roses. Postbloom dandelions are those magical puffy balls of seeds, which are often blown upon by daydreamers and the like—"I wish that Susie Thomas would have a crush on me!" Our stale breath and the wind often take these puffy seeds for a ride, dispersing them everywhere and turning that newly landscaped yard into a future dandelion bloom.

Dandelions are more than just free flowers; they are amazing health remedies. They can help promote digestion, stimulate the appetite, and increase the beneficial bacteria in your gut. If you need a diuretic, look no further! Dandelions are able to help the kidneys clear out waste, salt, and excess water by increasing urine production.

Dandelions have also been shown to improve liver function. But it doesn't stop there; this plant has been shown in research to slow cancer growth and prevent it from spreading (a claim not made lightly). It can also help regulate blood sugar and insulin levels, regulate blood pressure, regulate cholesterol levels, increase bile production in the gallbladder, reduce inflammation, and improve immunity. I think it's about time the dandelion gets its well-deserved praise. I love dandelion, as it's easy to grow (as seen on every high school soccer field) and for its wide range of uses. From salves to tinctures to teas, this herb should be in everyone's home.

The name dandelion comes from the French term *dent de lion*, meaning "tooth of the lion." These "weeds" have been used around the world for health purposes, with the dandelion root being the main source of medicinal value. In India and China, dandelion is used as a remedy for the liver. And while many people pay to have dandelions removed from their meticulously crafted gardens, these plants contain an immense array of vitamins and minerals. It has almost as much iron as spinach and up to four times the amount of vitamin A. The plant also has calcium, phosphorus, iron, magnesium, and sodium.

Health Benefits

HELPS PROTECT BONES

Dandelion is known to be high in calcium, an important mineral for your bones. Dandelion is also rich in antioxidants such as luteolin, which also protects bones from damage related to age.

Dandelions are also extremely high in vitamin K, another important vitamin for health and strong bones. Some say vitamin K is more important than calcium

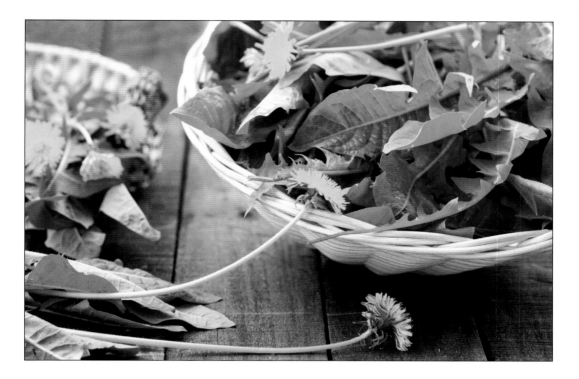

for bone strength and may reduce the risk of bone fractures in postmenopausal women who are at risk for osteoporosis. In fact, dandelion greens have 535 percent of the recommended daily value of vitamin K.

CLEANSES THE LIVER

In Chinese medicine, dandelion root is often used for the liver. Dandelions have been found to be useful at cleansing the liver and helping it work properly. They help with digestion by maintaining proper bile flow, which can help with constipation and prevent more serious gastrointestinal issues as well.

COMBATS DIABETES

Dandelion tea or juice might help people with diabetes due to its ability to keep blood sugar levels low by stimulating the production of insulin from the pancreas.

Dandelion tea is also able to help clear the body of excess sugar due to its diuretic properties. Be careful of drinking dandelion tea before bed; you'll get very acquainted with the bathroom in the middle of the night.

HIGH IN ANTIOXIDANTS

Dandelions are high in antioxidants, which help prevent certain cell damage and free radical damage. This is important, as it can be a key component in preventing cancer and other diseases. It might even be an antiaging remedy!

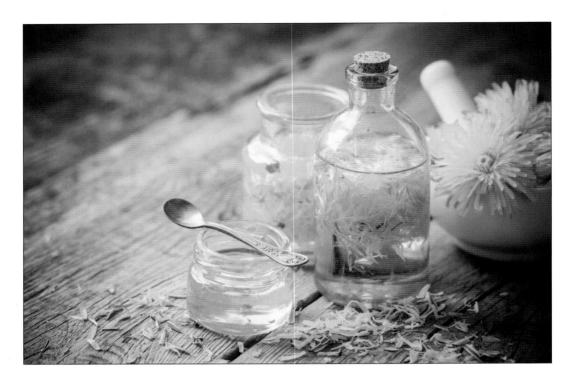

A study in 2011 at the University of Windsor in Canada found that dandelion root extract was effective in killing different cancers as a result of its free radical–killing abilities.[51]

PREVENTS URINARY TRACT INFECTIONS

It's been shown that dandelion root and leaf extracts from an herb called uva-ursi may reduce the number of urinary tract infections in women. The combination of the two herbs was able to kill bacteria, increase urine flow, and fight the infection.

Possible Side Effects, Contraindications, and Drug Interactions

Dandelion is generally considered safe. Some people have an allergic reaction from just touching the plant, and others may get mouth sores from ingesting it. In some people, dandelions may increase stomach acid and heartburn.

If you are allergic to ragweed, marigolds, chamomile, yarrow, daisies, or chrysanthemums, you should also avoid dandelion.

Those with kidney problems, gallbladder disease, or gallstones should consult their doctor before ingesting dandelion.

The dandelion leaf may act as a diuretic, which may make drugs leave your body faster. It can also interact with a number of medications that are broken down in the liver. If you are currently taking a prescription medication, consult your doctor before taking dandelion leaf. Medications that may interact with dandelion include antacids, blood-thinning medications, diuretics, lithium, ciprofloxacin, medications for diabetes, and medications broken down by the liver.

Dandelion Care Guide

While you could go ahead and just walk over to the nearest field and pick your dandelions for free, the bad news is that they're most likely contaminated with pesticides and other gross chemical contaminants. Believe me, you don't want to ingest that.

Growing dandelions from seed can be extremely easy and a great way to ensure you're not also eating chemical warfare designed to kill these amazing weeds. Simply buying dandelion seeds online and placing them in a pot is all you really have to do.

Pot: Buy a pot that is around six inches deep or deeper, with drainage holes.

Soil: Fill the container with all-purpose soil. Make sure the soil is moist before you spread the seeds. Sow the seeds about two to three inches apart. Don't cover the seeds with soil if you are growing them in a container. They'll grow best with a lot of exposed light.

Light: Light is important for the dandelion seeds to germinate and grow. Place the pot in a sunny, southward-facing window, or use grow lights.

Water: Water is also a valuable resource and you'll need plenty of it. Make sure you keep the soil moist at all times, but not overly wet. You don't want the soil to be soggy.

Your dandelions should reach maturity about two to three months after planting. If you decide you only want the baby dandelion greens and not the full plant, you can harvest your crop much sooner.

Reducing Bitterness: While bitter is a good thing, if you don't want your dandelion greens to be inedible, make sure to cover the plants with a dark fabric a few weeks before harvesting them. This will block out most of the light, which will reduce the bitterness while it blanches the leaves. The younger the leaves, the less bitter they'll be.

Harvesting Roots: There is no designated time to harvest dandelion roots.

Recipes and Remedies

Dandelion and Kale Salad

Eating dandelion leaves in a salad is one of the most delicious ways to gain the benefits of dandelion. The greens will give you 112 percent of your daily value of vitamin A as well as provide the wonderful vitamin K. The greens also have flavonoids such as zeaxanthin, carotene, lutein, and cryptoxanthin, which are known to protect the retina from ultraviolet rays and to protect the body from lung and mouth cancers.

Mixing dandelion greens with other greens, such as kale or spinach, will maximize the health benefits of the salad by a ton.

Ingredients:

- 1 cup dandelion greens
- 1 cup kale
- 2 teaspoons pumpkin seeds
- Any vegetable of your choice
- 2 tablespoons olive oil
- 1 tablespoon vinegar

Instructions:

Chop the dandelion greens and mix together with other ingredients in a large bowl. Toss the salad in the olive oil and vinegar and enjoy!

Dandelion Root Tea or Coffee

Dandelion coffee or tea can be an amazing option for those trying to quit their coffee and caffeine addictions. This savory, nutty, dark drink definitely looks the part, and tastes even better. Not to mention, you're gaining a ton of health benefits from this delicious drink without all the jitters and shaky hands.

Ingredients:

- 1 cup chopped dandelion roots

Instructions:

1. Preheat your oven to 250°F. Put your dandelion roots on a cookie sheet and leave them in the oven for two to three hours, until they are completely dry.
2. Grind your roots in a mortar and pestle. Store them in a cool and dark place.

3. Make your tea using a tea infuser or something similar. Steep the roots in the hot water for around three minutes, and then separate out.
4. Enjoy! You can add any additions to your tea, such as cream, butter, or honey.

Dandelion Wine

Dandelion wine has been around for centuries, with countless generations of people getting drunk off this yellow concoction. It is the Europeans who created the recipe, aptly naming it the "cheap man's wine," and recipes of this unique beverage have been passed down as a family tradition in a surprising number of homes. Try this medicinal liquor yourself, and gain some health benefits while you sip on your nightcap. Like brewing beer or making your own "real" wine, dandelion wine is not for the faint of heart. You'll need some dedication and perseverance, but if you have what it takes, it might be the next best thing added to your liquor cabinet.

Ingredients:

- 230 grams whole dandelion flowers (if you want a wine that is less bitter, use just the petals)
- ¼ cup warm water (for soaking)
- 4 quarts water
- 3 tablespoons lime juice

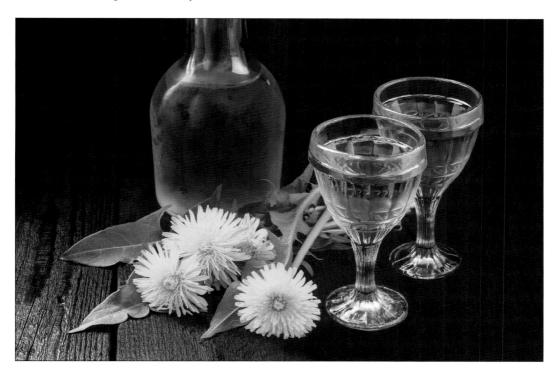

- 1 cup orange juice
- 3 tablespoons lemon juice
- ½ teaspoon powdered ginger
- 3 tablespoons chopped orange zest
- 1 tablespoon chopped lemon zest
- 6 cups sugar
- 8 whole cloves
- 1 package dried brewing yeast
- Glass wine bottles
- Corks

Instructions:

1. Gather your dandelion flowers and wash them thoroughly. Make sure to get rid of all the green material.
2. Soak your flowers for two days in water.
3. Once soaked, put your blossoms in 4 quarts of water and combine with the lime, orange, and lemon juices.
4. Stir in your ginger, orange and lemon zests, sugar, and cloves.
5. Bring the mix to a slow boil for an hour.
6. Strain the mixture through coffee filters and let the infusion cool down.
7. Stir in the yeast while the infusion is still warm, but below 100°F.
8. Cover the mixture and leave it overnight.
9. The next day, pour the mixture into glass wine bottles.
10. Cork your bottles once the mixture has been poured into them.
11. Store the bottles in a dark place and let ferment for up to a month.

This recipe will start as an experiment and end as a family recipe. Everyone puts their own spin on dandelion wine, and it's meant for playful experimentation. See what added spices you like, try more bitter or sweeter versions, or decide if you want to ferment longer or shorter.

Dandelion Abscess Poultice

Dandelions have been used for thousands of years to help treat abscesses, sores, eczema, psoriasis, rashes, and other joyless bodily manifestations we'd rather not talk about. Creating a dandelion-based poultice is a great way to heal and resolve these nasty issues. Poultices are topical applications typically made from herbs. Making poultices is simple, cost-effective, and fun, utilizing the amazing herbal remedies you have growing in your home.

This dandelion poultice is great to use on the skin for a variety of skin issues, such as itchy and dry skin, acne, eczema, rashes, and even bruises. Similar to

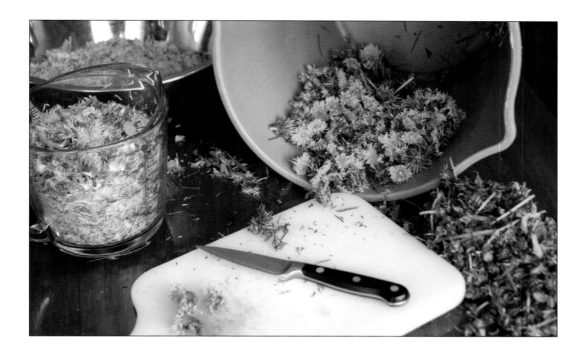

making a mojito, you'll want to take out your mortar and pestle and get your muscles working, as you'll need to crush the herbs into a paste. Making a poultice doesn't have to be a chore; it's as simple as gathering your fresh leaves and chopping. The amount of herbs you use is up to you; it depends on how much of the skin needs to be covered.

Ingredients:

- Fresh dandelion leaves
- Mortar and pestle or blender

Instructions:

1. Take the dandelion leaves and chop them into small pieces, then transfer to a mortar and pestle to further crush the herbs until they become a pulp. The end result doesn't have to be perfectly smooth and silky, just crushed with the juices flowing.
2. If you like, place the herbs in a blender or food processor to get the same results.
3. Spread the crushed herbs on the area of skin which needs to be covered. Cover with gauze or muslin to hold the poultice in place. To relieve symptoms, you can leave the poultice on overnight or throughout the day.

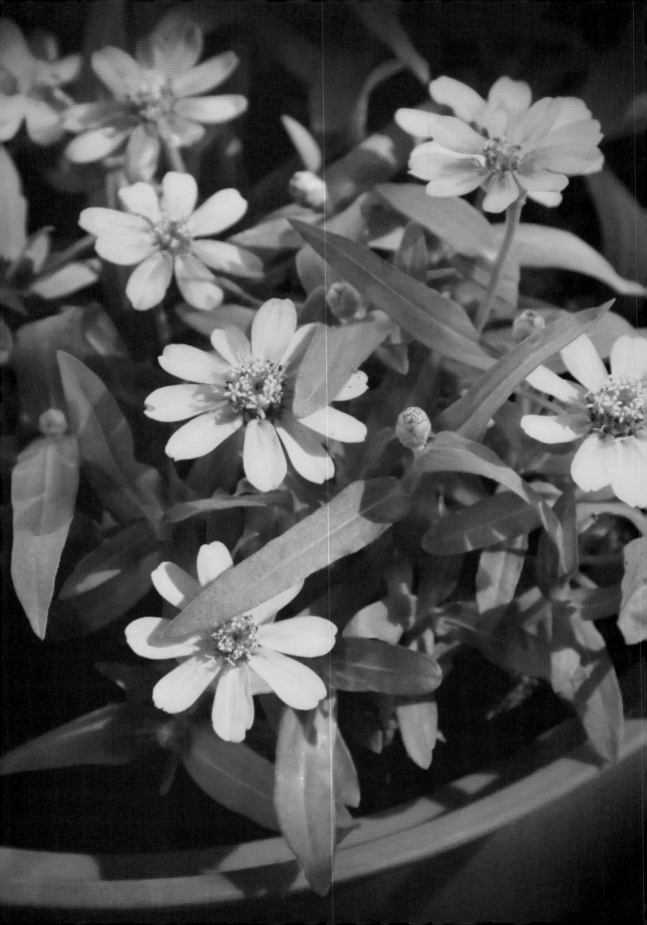

Chapter Ten: Calendula

Calendula officinalis

Also known as pot marigolds, calendula plants are beautiful, edible flowers that are reliable and easy to grow. However, don't get them confused with the common marigold, as they are not in the same genus. Native to the Mediterranean, the calendula is now grown everywhere for its ornamental value and its ability to attract bees for pollination while keeping harmful insects away from other plants. Brought to North America by early settlers, the word *calendula* comes from the Latin *calens*, meaning "the first day of each month" because the Romans believed they bloomed the first day of every month. The calendula plant was a symbol of joy, bringing nonstop happiness to everyone through its nonstop blooming nature. The term *marigold* comes from the Christian religion, as the plant bloomed at all the festivals celebrating the Virgin Mary.

Historical uses of this herb are numerous, including being used as an aphrodisiac. In the middle ages, wearing marigolds around your neck would give you visions of anyone who had robbed you, and an old legend believed that if maidens

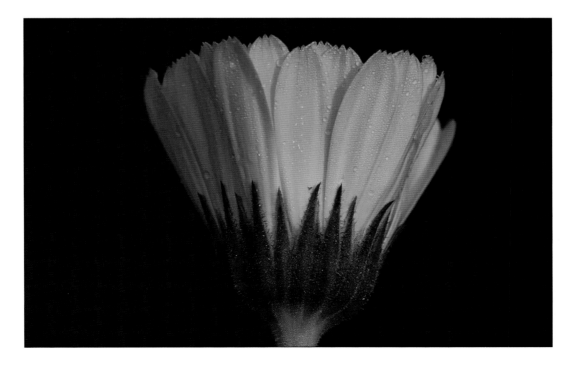

touched marigolds with their bare feet, they would understand the language of birds. During the American Civil War, doctors used the flowers to treat open wounds on the battlefield, as they were effective antiseptics, preventing infection and staunching the bleeding. Doctors continued to use marigolds through World War II.

Today, the calendula is used for its wide range of healing qualities. This plant is essential for every beginner gardener, not just for the appeal of easy care, but for their immense health benefits. The beautiful orange flowers have a slight honey aroma and are edible delicacies often used as garnish. The petals themselves contain a wide array of health benefits, including high levels of antioxidants such as carotenoids and flavonoids, and they also contain lutein and beta-carotene, which are both absorbed and converted into vitamin A by the body.

This plant is medicine, able to heal wounds, treat digestive issues and ulcers, relieve menstrual cramps, fight fungal infections, reduce inflammation, and rid you from potential viruses. This herb is a wonderful remedy for women, and drinking calendula tea on a regular basis can help reduce painful periods, regulate menstrual bleeding, and balance hormones. Calendula can be made into creams, oils, gels, tinctures, teas, or compresses.

Health Benefits

ANTI-INFLAMMATORY PROPERTIES

Every herb in this book has anti-inflammatory properties, which should scream to you the importance of eating your plants and herbs. Calendula, however, has very strong anti-inflammatory abilities, containing powerful and healthful substances known as flavonoids. Flavonoids are able to protect cells from free radical damage as well as C-reactive protein and cytokenes. This correlates into an incredible ability to prevent cancer and other chronic illnesses.

Linoleic acid, which is found in high amounts in the calendula plant, has been known to treat a wide range of ailments, including ear infections, sore throats, diaper rash, ulcers, and more. In fact, you can find some ear drop solutions in the store containing calendula.

AIDS SKIN HEALTH

Due to its rich nature in antioxidants, vitamin A precursors, and vitamin E, calendula is an easy choice when it comes to your skin. Calendula is able to soften the skin; reduce signs of aging; treat burns, skin infections, dermatitis, dry skin, eczema, and insect bites; and more. There are even some studies which suggest calendula can increase collagen production, a protein important for elasticity, firmness, and integrity. Improving your collagen production means younger-looking skin and a younger-looking you.

HEALS ULCERS AND HEMORRHOIDS

It's been shown in some research that calendula is able to increase the speed of healing in slow-healing wounds, as well as improve blood flow and oxygen to infected areas as well as wounds. This increased blood flow and oxygen help the body grow new tissue and heal faster.[52] This is also why calendula is helpful for ulcers.

REGULATE MENSTRUATION

If you're a woman who dreads her monthly visit from "Aunt Flo," there's good news. Drinking calendula tea can help regulate the menstrual cycle, decreasing those painful cramps. Due to the high amounts of flavonoids, the herb helps to relax the muscles, allowing for a more pain-free existence.

ANTIVIRAL AND ANTIBACTERIAL

Calendula is such a powerful antibacterial and antiviral herb that it was used on the battlefields of both World War I and World War II. The antimicrobial effect of calendula is enhanced with the addition of sunflower oil, due to its linoleic and oleic acid content.[53]

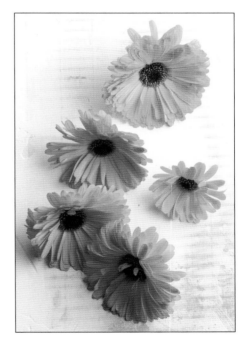

Possible Side Effects, Contraindications, and Drug Interactions

Calendula is generally considered safe; however, under no circumstances should it be applied to an open wound without a doctor's supervision.

If you are allergic to plants in the daisy family, which includes chrysanthemums, ragweed, daisies, and more, you should also avoid calendula, as it can cause a skin rash.

Pregnant and breastfeeding women should not use calendula. Additionally, those trying to conceive should avoid use of calendula, as it could potentially cause miscarriage.

Calendula should be used with caution when combined with sedatives, medications to treat high blood pressure, and medications used to treat diabetes.

Calendula Care Guide

Calendula is a beautiful plant to grow indoors, one which will give you a constant state of blooms and bright-orange hues to brighten your home. Outside, these plants can grow up to two feet tall, and flowers tend to open when the sun is out and the weather is dry. They'll often close when the weather is cold or moist. Indoors, calendula plants may not grow as tall, but they'll be perfectly happy in a pot in a sunny window.

Light: Calendulas prefer full sun. Make sure to place them in a southward-facing window, and place outdoors in the warmer months.

Water: Keep the soil evenly moist, and use warm water. As usual, don't overwater or let them sit in water.

Soil: Rich, well-drained soil.

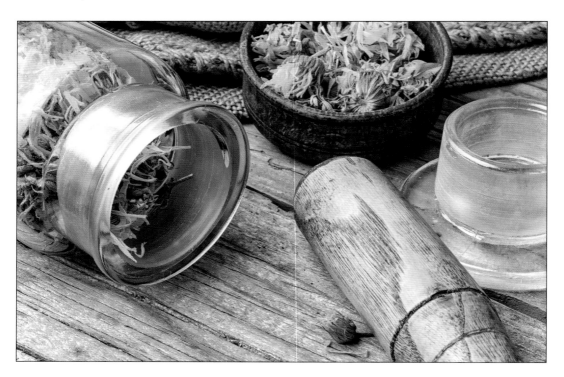

Recipes and Remedies

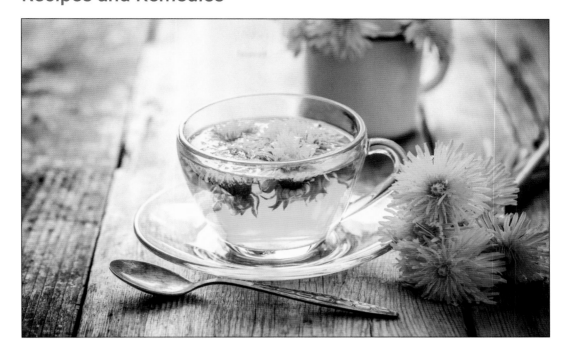

Calendula Tea for Urinary Tract Infections

Tea made from calendula is a great option for the treatment of urinary tract infections, those amazing reminders of womanhood which make you want to urinate every five minutes for days on end. If you are someone prone to these infections, drinking this tea on a regular basis can help prevent future occurrences.

The tea is also beneficial for those with sore throats, providing a soothing feeling to a sore and itchy throat, as well as aiding digestion, helping with canker sores or mouth ulcers, and more.

Making tea from your own flowers is an extremely easy way to attain major health benefits from your indoor plants. Just dry your flowers and steep them in hot water. Done!

Ingredients:

- Small handful of dried calendula blossoms
- Hot water

Instructions:

1. Simply pour boiling water over your dried calendula blossoms and steep for fifteen minutes.
2. After fifteen minutes, strain off the flowers and drink your tea!

Calendula Facial Toner

Calendula makes a fantastic facial toner for its abilities to help soothe the skin, reduce inflammation, and help heal wounds and skin irritations. Using a calendula facial toner will help your skin smooth out, have fewer blemishes, and get rid of those annoying skin irritations. Use this toner not only on your face but on any part of the skin that has any rashes or irritations you want to reduce. This is an extremely easy and useful toner to make, with hardly any prep time needed.

Ingredients:

- ¼ cup dried calendula flowers
- 6 ounces distilled water
- 1 tablespoon aloe juice

Instructions:

1. Make an herbal tea using your dried calendula flowers and distilled water. Let the tea steep for twenty minutes.
2. Strain your herbs.
3. Add 1 tablespoon of aloe juice to your tea. Place the concoction in a bottle and label it.

Calendula Lip Balm

For those who suffer from never-ending chapped lips, ditch the toxic, expensive, menthol lip options at the pharmacy. Why not create your own natural, skin-loving lip balm at home? This recipe will help moisten the lips while also helping your chapped skin and caring for your wounded lips.

Ingredients:

- 2 tablespoons calendula-infused olive oil (Follow recipe for Lavender Oil on page 58, except use calendula blossoms instead of lavender.)
- 4 tablespoons beeswax
- 6 tablespoons calendula-infused coconut oil (Follow recipe for Lavender Oil on page 58, except use calendula blossoms instead of lavender and use coconut oil as the carrier oil.)
- 1 teaspoon vitamin E oil
- 10 drops lavender essential oil
- 5 drops peppermint essential oil
- Lip balm tubes

Instructions:

1. In a double boiler, mix together your olive oil, beeswax, and coconut oil. If you don't have a double boiler, you can make your own by placing a bowl in a shallow pan of water.
2. Wait until your beeswax has melted and then remove from the heat. Stir in the vitamin E and your essential oils.
3. Once everything is mixed, start filling your lip balm tubes.
4. Once filled, let them sit and cool. You can place the tubes in the refrigerator to expedite the process. Once the mixture is cool, place the lids on the tubes.

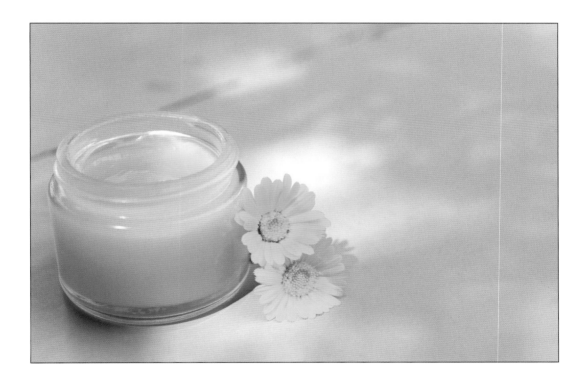

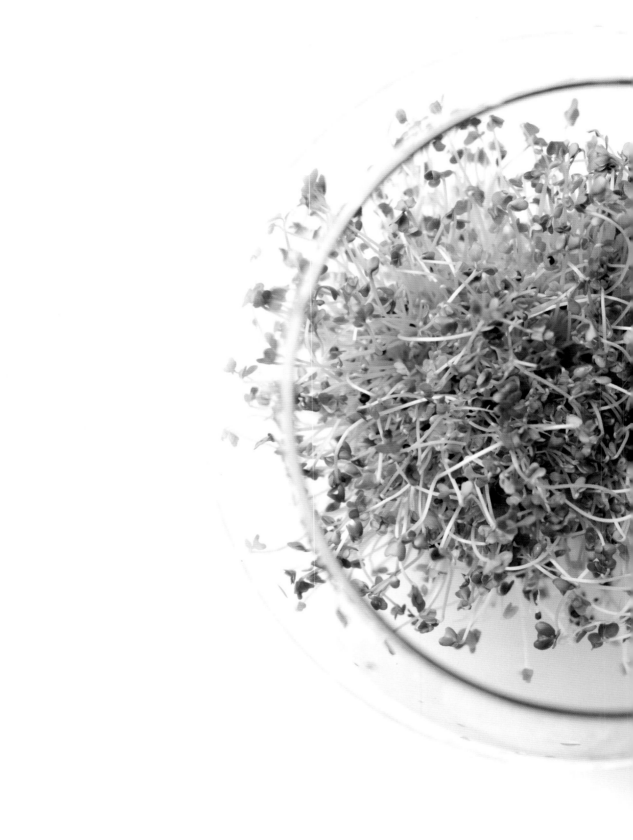

Chapter Eleven:
Broccoli Sprouts

Brassica oleracea

Not necessarily known as a popular houseplant, broccoli sprouts are fun and easy to grow in the home for a unique experience—think chia pets, but healthier and not as creepy. While you won't grow them for how they'll look on your windowsill, broccoli sprouts are a purely utilitarian approach to indoor gardening, as they'll spend most of their time inside a dark cabinet and then immediately be thrown into your belly.

Broccoli sprouts are some of the healthiest foods you can eat on earth. In fact, they provide so many health benefits, when reading up on them, you may feel like you're in the middle of a late night QVC ad. From cancer prevention to fighting depression, diabetes, aging, heart disease, respiratory disease, gastric diseases, and even autism, broccoli sprouts may be the miracle food you've never heard of.

Broccoli sprouts are one hundred times higher in some cancer-fighting compounds than the actual mature vegetable (broccoli), and contain a magic ingredient—sulforaphane (SFN)—a powerful anticancer compound that helps fight and reduce the risk of developing cancer. SFN is one of the most well-researched chemicals on earth, and is becoming increasingly popular due to its incredible healing abilities. And while you could eat pounds and pounds of kale, mature broccoli, and Brussels sprouts to get the benefits of SFN, eating just a few ounces of broccoli sprouts offer the same benefits. In fact, broccoli sprouts have the highest concentration of SFN around.

But the healing benefits of broccoli sprouts don't just end at SFN; they also contain other incredible compounds such as indole-3-carbinol, carotenoids, kaempferol, quercetin, and many vitamins, including vitamin C, vitamin K1, potassium, folate, iron, and magnesium.

Sprouts are easy to grow and fun to have around the kitchen—putting a handful every morning in your daily smoothie, placing it on top of your favorite salad, or adding a dash to garnish your favorite soup. Adding broccoli sprouts to your daily routine can completely transform your health, helping prevent an array of chronic disease, reduce body fat, and energize you for the day.

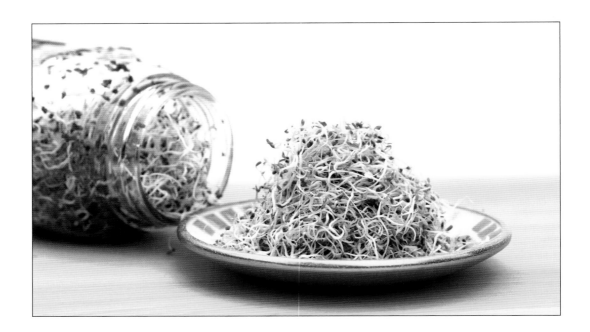

Health Benefits

ABOUT SULFORAPHANE (SFN)

A phytochemical found in cruciferous vegetables, SFN is the magic word these days, with bloggers, nutrition experts, doctors, and other nutrition gurus raving about its massive list of health benefits. This magical ingredient is known as an isothiocyanate, a sulfur-containing compound, and is activated while chewing your food, cutting your food, or "disrupting" the plant. To get more detailed, crushing or chewing the sprouts activates an enzyme called myrosinase, which converts compounds called glucosinolates into isothiocyanates. Still with me?

In short, make sure you don't just swallow the sprouts whole; chew on those lucious greens with everything you've got, and swallow it down knowing you're getting the most incredible health supplement on earth. Soak in that health! Its ability to boost the antioxidant capacity of cells, and its power to promote detoxification, is one of the main reasons researchers believe SFN to be so incredibly beneficial and potent.

It's been shown that three-day-old sprouts can contain up to one hundred times the amount of the SFN precursor, glucoraphanin, than mature plants. And raw broccoli sprouts have the highest amount of glucoraphanin, and thus SFN, out there.

While supplement companies are competing to come up with the most bioavailable and potent SFN-containing supplement out there, nothing beats eating raw, organic broccoli sprouts. While the list of health benefits stemming from

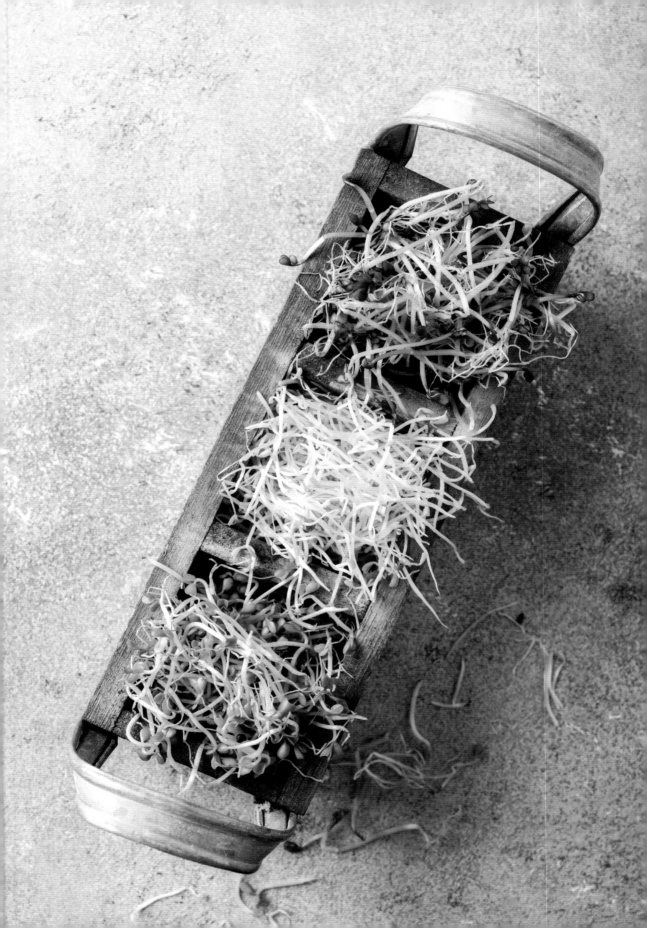

SFN is seemingly endless, here is my attempt to write about the most interesting benefits. Good luck to all of us.

PREVENTS AND COMBATS CANCER

One of the most researched and exciting possibilities of SFN is its potential to prevent and combat cancer. Out of the thousands of compounds found in plants that are able to prevent and kill cancer, SFN is by far one of the most promising. Not only has it been shown to kill cancer cells, but it has very little effect on healthy cells. SFN also has been shown to reduce DNA damage and mutation rates when cancer-causing chemicals bind to DNA, thus keeping us healthy from our toxic lives.[54]

And SFN is indiscriminatory when it comes to cancer. It has been shown to kill colorectal cancer, oral squamous cell carcinoma, breast cancer cells, cervical cancer cells, and liver, prostate, and leukemia cells as well. Working from various angles, SFN is able to not only induce cell cancer death but prevent cancer genes from activating, eliminate DNA damage, and inhibit enzymes that can activate procarcinogens. This stuff is amazing.

What's more, SFN has been shown to enhance the efficacy of cancer drugs, making them work better and reducing their toxicity on healthy cells.

COMBAT DIABETES

You read that right: just adding a daily serving of broccoli sprouts may improve outcomes of people with diabetes.[55] SFN has been shown to increase HDL cholesterol while decreasing triglycerides, oxidative stress, C-reactive protein, and insulin. It's also been shown to prevent diabetes-related complications such as neuropathy, tissue damage, heart damage, and more.

LOWERS CHOLESTEROL

Eating broccoli sprouts has been shown to reduce LDL cholesterol in humans. One study had participants eat one hundred grams of sprouts per day for one week, and their LDL cholesterol decreased while their HDL cholesterol increased.[56]

DECREASES CARDIOVASCULAR DISEASE

If your family has a history of heart disease, it may be time to start eating your sprouts. SFN has been shown to prevent and combat cardiovascular disease. It's also shown that a diet high in glucoraphanin decreases blood pressure, while protecting the heart against oxidative stress and reducing heart damage after an infarct.[57]

The magic of SFN doesn't stop there; it's also been shown to protect against the hardening of arteries and to decrease inflammation in hardened arteries, while reducing blood clot formation. SFN decreases the amount of damaged tissue from a stroke and maintains neurological function after a stroke.

BOOSTS THE IMMUNE SYSTEM

Stop getting sick every flu season and start bingeing on broccoli sprouts. SFN increases the activity of natural killer cells, which enables your body to rid itself of those annoying bacterial infections.[58] Even more, it's been shown that SFN boosts immunity in aging mice.

ANTIVIRAL, ANTIBACTERIAL, AND ANTIFUNGAL

Eating broccoli sprouts will enhance your antiviral response, specifically having significant antiviral activity against the flu, HIV, Epstein-Barr, and hepatitis C.[59]

One study has shown SFN to inhibit twenty-three out of twenty-eight bacterial and fungal species tested.[60]

PROTECTS THE SKIN FROM SUN DAMAGE

No, we're not asking you to generously rub broccoli sprouts all over your body. In fact, ingesting them will be enough. It's been found that our favorite compound, SFN, has been shown to protect against UVA and UVB radiation, sunburn, and subsequent skin damage, so you don't have to stop falling asleep at the beach just yet.[61]

Three-day-old broccoli sprouts have been shown to protect against UV radiation–induced inflammation and to help stop redness. They also protect against oxidative stress caused by UVA radiation, which has been known to play a role in the premature aging and weathering of skin, reducing the body's ability to create collagen. SFN also helps alleviate any blistering of the skin caused by sun radiation.

COMBATS DEPRESSION AND ANXIETY

Recent research has shown depression to be a form of inflammation in the body. Increased inflammation can be a major contributing factor to anxiety and depression, and broccoli sprouts have been shown to help combat these symptoms.

In clinical trials, mice that have repeated ingestion of SFN reverse their depression and anxiety-like behaviors.[62] This is likely due to an inhibition of the hypothalamic-pituitary-adrenal axis and the inflammatory response to stress.

RESTORES COGNITIVE FUNCTION

One of the most exciting aspects of SFN is its potential to help restore cognitive function.[63] Studies have shown that SFN increases neuronal brain-derived neurotrophic factor, a protein that has been shown to play an important role in neuroplasticity, the ability of the brain to form new connections and form new neurons and synapses during the learning process or following an injury.

SFN also reduces inflammation in the brain, which may help in cases of neurodegenerative disorders. SFN has been shown to help improve cognitive performance after traumatic brain injury, increase memory, and protect neurons against neurotoxicity. And this is just the beginning.

MAY HELP WITH PARKINSON'S DISEASE

Some studies show SFN being beneficial with those suffering from Parkinson's disease.[64] In animal models, SFN inhibits dopaminergic neuronal loss (a hallmark of Parkinson's) and can improve deficits in motor coordination.

MAY HELP WITH ALZHEIMER'S DISEASE

Broccoli sprouts won't just help with traumatic brain injuries but also with neurodegenerative brain diseases like Alzheimer's.[65] SFN reduces the production of what's known as amyloid beta, a peptide which is a major factor implicated in the formation of Alzheimer's. Also, SFN reduces plaque formations of amyloid beta as well as reducing neuron loss, while improving cognitive impairment.

MAY HELP WITH AUTISM

Autism rates are increasing worldwide, with numerous theories as to why this is occurring and how to help treat the symptoms. One of the treatments is an addition of broccoli sprouts to the diet. A small study found that SFN helped improve symptoms in two-thirds of those who took a supplement.[66] The study looked at the effects of SFN on twenty-six men with moderate to severe autism for eighteen weeks. Improvements were seen in irritability, lethargy, awareness, communication, motivation, and mannerisms. While this is a small study, it shows promise for further investigations into the effect of SFN on autism.

MAY BE BENEFICIAL FOR SUBSTANCE ABUSE

For those suffering with substance abuse, the road to recovery may seem long and unattainable. However, there may be some help simply from eating sprouted broccoli. It's been shown that SFN can improve behavioral changes associated with methamphetamine exposure in mice.[67] Pretreating the mice with SFN attenuated increased movement in mice after a single dose of methamphetamine.[68]

Can Improve Digestion and Gastrointestinal Inflammation

SFN is able to protect the gut against NSAIDs, our favorite painkillers. NSAIDs, such as [advil is a brand name for ibuprofen] ibuprofen, have been shown to cause a range of side effects, including stomach pains and ulcers, liver or kidney problems, high blood pressure, and more. SFN may help combat these effects by inhibiting gastric ulcers in rats, preventing aspirin-related injury to the gut, and reducing inflammation.

Protects the Liver

Worried about your liver? Eat broccoli sprouts. Broccoli sprouts improved liver function in men with fatty liver disease and in animals.[69] SFN protected against numerous liver diseases caused by toxicity, drugs, and alcohol.[70, 71, 72]

Reduces Damage from Pollution

If you live in a big city, especially one that is known for its smog, eating broccoli sprouts can help prevent potential health damage from pollution. Broccoli sprouts aid the body in detoxifying pollutants such as pesticides, heavy metals, and airborne toxins by activating detoxification systems and can decrease the risk of developing certain cancers.[73]

If you're a smoker, you should be eating broccoli sprouts every day, as they will induce phase II enzymes in the upper airways and help protect you against the numerous toxins in cigarettes.

SFN also helps protect human white blood cells from pesticide-induced DNA damage for those who live near or on nonorganic farms, or just anyone who gets their lawn sprayed.[74]

May Combat Asthma

For those suffering from asthma, start stocking up on broccoli sprout seeds and get to eating. Sprouts have been shown to benefit animals with asthma and to reduce airway inflammation.[75] They also have been shown to help reduce airway inflammation in humans who have been exposed to diesel exhaust particles. Research is still new regarding asthma, and some studies have shown no improvements with asthma or Chronic Obstructive Pulmonary Disease (COPD) symptoms.

Possible Side Effects, Contraindications, and Drug Interactions

Broccoli sprouts are generally considered safe. However, sprouts in general may carry bacteria that may cause illness when eaten. Make sure your seeds are clean before sprouting.

If you are allergic or sensitive to broccoli or other members of the cruciferous, cabbage, or mustard family, stay away.

Pregnant and breastfeeding women should avoid eating broccoli sprouts due to the possible bacteria.

Broccoli sprouts may cause lowered blood pressure, so caution is urged for those who are currently taking other drugs or supplements to lower blood pressure.

Use caution if you are taking cholesterol-lowering drugs.

SFN, the active ingredient in broccoli sprouts, may interfere with how the body processes certain drugs and herbs which use the liver's cytochrome P450 enzyme system. As a result, the levels of drugs or supplements may be increased in the blood and can cause an increase in the effect or a potentially serious adverse reaction.

Broccoli Sprout Care Guide

Sprouts are incredibly easy to grow in your home year-round, with little fuss and low-cost maintenance. Just throw those seeds in a mason jar and you're all set! Well, almost. While it's super easy to grow sprouts at home, be careful to keep your hands clean, as well as the jar and other surfaces—they are more easily contaminated than other types of greens.

Ingredients:

- 3 tablespoons organic broccoli sprout seeds
- Wide-mouth mason jar
- Water
- Sprouting lid

Instructions:

1. Take 3 tablespoons of broccoli sprout seeds and place them in a mason jar.
2. Pour warm, purified water into the jar, making sure it just covers the seeds.
3. Let seeds soak overnight in a warm and dark place. I like soaking them in a kitchen cabinet.
4. After eight to ten hours, drain off the water and rinse the seeds with warm and fresh water. After rinsing, make sure to drain off the water again, vigorously shaking the jar to get as much of the water out as possible.
5. Place the mason jar on its side in a bowl with the sprouting lid down so the water can drain off. Place it in a cabinet.

6. Rinse the seeds two to three times per day for around four to five days.
7. Watch the seeds begin to sprout and grow!
8. Once your sprouts are a few centimeters long and have defined yellow tails, move your jar out near exposed sunlight. I usually place mine on a windowsill. Allow the sprouts to use the light to grow quickly. Be sure to keep rinsing the sprouts so they don't dry out.
9. The sprouts will be ready to eat once they have darker green leaves and are about an inch or longer in length.

How Many Sprouts Should You Eat Per Day?

According to Dr. Rhonda Patrick, a doctor in biomedical science and an expert in nutrition, eating around 100–140 grams of sprouts per day will yield enough SFN to equal what researchers use in studies. This is easy to calculate simply by getting a kitchen scale and weighing out your daily portions.

If you feel like this is too much to eat per day, eating any amount will surely boost your health. Making sure to eat them on a regular basis will be the most important gauge of whether or not you will gain any benefits from ingesting them.

How to Maximize SFN in Your Broccoli Sprouts

If you truly want to maximize the benefits of your sprouts, make sure to follow a few steps. First, heating your broccoli sprouts by boiling, baking, or sautéing them in butter will only decrease the amount of SFN in your magical meal. Instead, eat your sprouts raw, in a smoothie or on a salad, to obtain full benefits.

Another trick to boost your SFN even more is to add a pinch of mustard seed. Mustard seed is a myrosinase-containing food, which means it can boost the SFN formation in your sprouts. A study found that participants who ate a broccoli supplement without active myrosinase had significantly lower levels of SFN than those that did eat broccoli (any type) with mustard seed.

If you feel like you must sauté or boil your sprouts or mature broccoli, make sure you add a pinch of mustard seed to those greens. The same goes for eating frozen broccoli, which typically has a reduced amount of myrosinase, as it's been blanched as a part of the processing.

Recipes

Longevity Broccoli Smoothie

Smoothies are always a great way to gulp down nutrition, making them an easy and ideal breakfast or meal on the go. However, let's be real. Broccoli sprouts aren't the most amazing-tasting food on earth. Their earthy, dirt-like taste can stick in your mouth long after you chew them, or drink them. Blending them with berries and coconut milk helps to disguise their strong flavor, while adding more nutrients to your smoothie.

Ingredients:

- 50 grams broccoli sprouts
- 1 cup coconut milk or alternatives
- ¼ cup blueberries

Instructions:

1. Place all ingredients in a blender and blend, making sure the blueberries and sprouts are ground.
2. Add extra coconut milk to desired consistency.

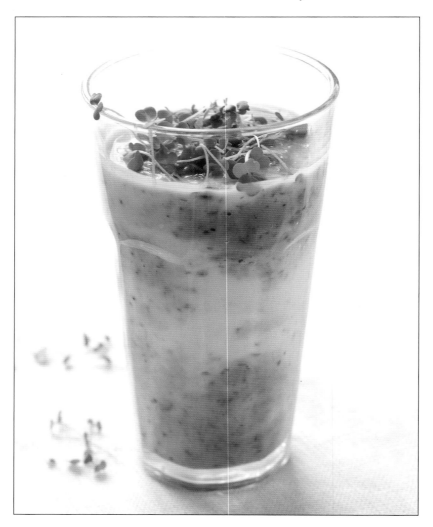

Broccoli Sprout Dip

This powerhouse dip is perfect with chips, crackers, or crudites.

Ingredients:

- ¼ cup raw pumpkin seeds, soaked in spring water for two hours
- ¾ cup raw cashews
- ½ cup yellow bell pepper, washed, deseeded, and chopped
- 3 tablespoons freshly squeezed lemon juice
- 1 clove garlic, peeled and crushed
- ½ tablespoon fresh turmeric (curcumin) or ¾ tablespoon turmeric powder
- ½ tablespoon fresh or ½ teaspoon dried oregano
- ½ cup spring or filtered water
- ¼ cup broccoli sprouts, rinsed and cut in half
- ½ cup fresh dill, rinsed and chopped
- 2 tablespoons cold-pressed organic hemp seed oil
- Pink or sea salt to taste

Instructions:

1. Blend all the ingredients and spices except the broccoli sprouts, dill, and hemp seed oil until smooth.
2. Add remaining ingredients to the mixture above. Pulse or blend on low until the oil and fresh greens are finely chopped but still visible.
3. Adjust the seasoning to taste and enjoy. This will last for up to a week in the refrigerator.

Adding sprouts to your meals every day is easy and delicious. You don't need a recipe; just toss a handful of broccoli sprouts in your salad, place them on your sandwich, eat them with your eggs, blend them with your smoothies, and more. Broccoli sprouts can be the easiest and healthiest food you add to your routine ever. Don't like the taste? Toss them in olive oil and vinegar, or just add butter. Butter makes everything taste better.

There is no reason to delay eating sprouts, so buy some seeds online, get your mason jars in order, and start sprouting. The immense healing benefits rival blockbuster drugs, and there are no side effects. If you want to be healthier, feel better, and stay on a budget, there is no better way to get on track than with broccoli sprouts.

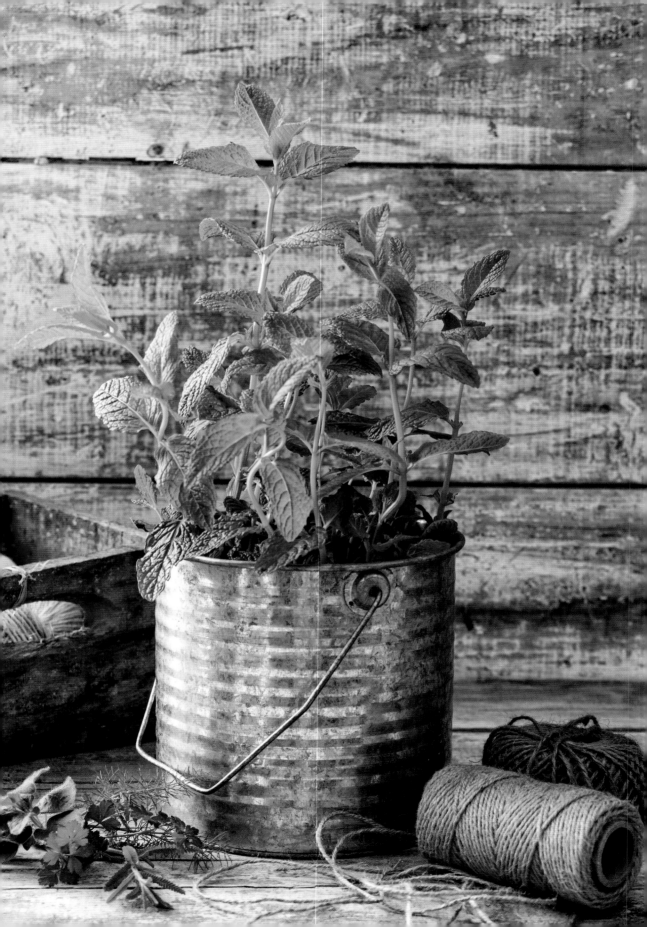

Chapter Twelve: Mint

Mentha

One of the best-known herbs in the world, mint can be used to help promote digestion, reduce inflammation, and soothe the stomach. Mint has one of the highest antioxidant capacities of any food, tastes delicious, and is easy to grow. In fact, mint is so easy to grow, many people find it grows too well in their gardens. It grows easily and spreads quickly.

Used for centuries as a gastrointestinal aid, at least thirteen species are distributed across North America, Europe, Asia, Australia, and Africa. Mint is a perennial herb whose name comes from Greek mythology, referring to a nymph named Minthe or Menthe and who, according to legend, was Pluto's girlfriend. According to the myth, Pluto's wife, Persephone, became jealous and turned Minthe into a ground-clinging plant. And while Pluto wasn't able to rescue

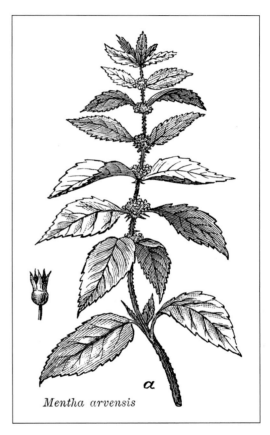

Mentha arvensis

his girlfriend from the plant she had become, he decided to give her the ability of sweetening the air when her leaves were crushed. How romantic!

While mint is widely used today for its culinary prowess, it's still commonly utilized for its health benefits. In Chinese medicine, mint, also known as "Bo He," is considered to have pungent, aromatic, and cool properties. It's often used to treat diarrhea and painful menstruation, clear up rashes, and more. The German Commission E has approved the internal use of mint for many conditions such as gastrointestinal issues, gallbladder disorders, and flatulence, and even for external use for neuralgia.

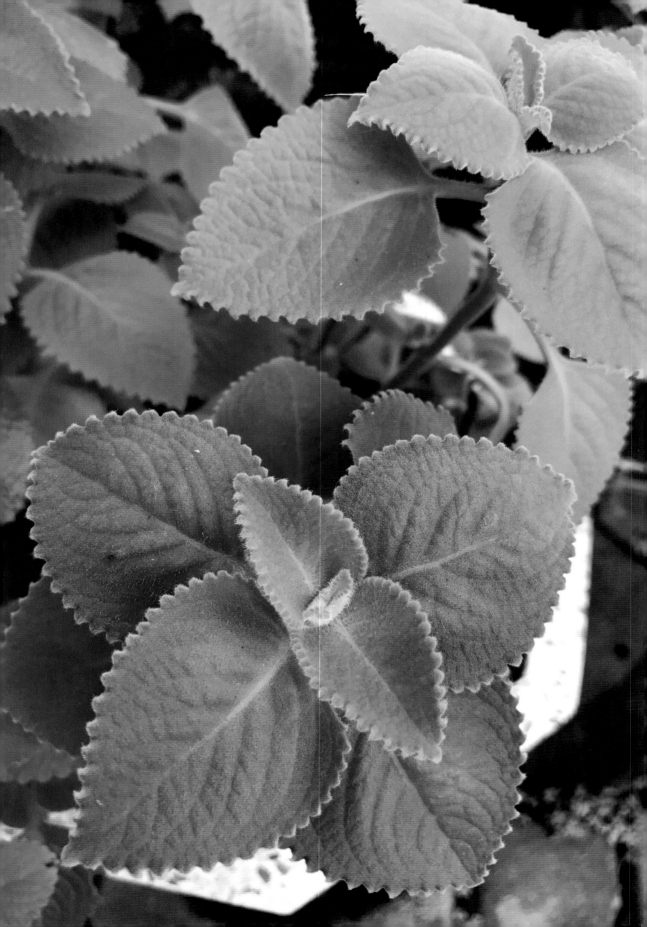

Health Benefits

HELPS BREASTFEEDING

For women trying to breastfeed, peppermint water may be effective in preventing nipple cracks and nipple pain for first-time mothers. While breastfeeding is an optimal method to feed your child, it's not necessarily kind to a new mother's breasts. Sipping mint-infused water can be the difference between painful and sore nipples and smooth sailing.

EASES COMMON COLDS

What do Vicks VapoRub and your favorite cold remedies have in common? Menthol. Menthol is found in mint and is a natural decongestant that can break up mucus, phlegm, and other annoying side effects of the common cold. Peppermint tea has been shown to relieve a sore throat, and making your own vapor rub can be a nontoxic alternative to store-bought remedies.

AIDS DIGESTION

If you have an upset stomach, start eating more mint. Mint may increase and encourage bile flow, which helps make your digestion move quicker and smoother. And if you run on the bloaty, gassy side of things, mint may help relieve pain and discomfort from your "windy" days.

COMBATS IBS

If you're one of the twenty-five to forty-four million people in the United States suffering from IBS, it might be a good time to start growing mint in your backyard. Peppermint oil has been found to be an effective remedy for those who have abdominal pain and discomfort associated with IBS. One study found that those who took enteric-coated peppermint oil capsules twice a day for four weeks had a 50 percent reduction in total IBS symptoms.

SOOTHES SKIN

If you've been bitten by any bug you know the annoying and frustrating itching and burning associated with these unfortunate side effects of outdoor living. But don't fret; mint can be your next best friend. Using a mint lotion can have a cooling effect on the skin, which can ease pain, redness, and swelling associated with insect bites. Hallelujah.

EASES PAIN

Got pain? No worries. For all those who whimper with every sore muscle, applying peppermint extract to areas of pain has been found to increase the pain threshold in humans, allowing you to endure more pain and suffer less.

RELIEVES NAUSEA AND HEADACHES

Freshly crushed mint leaves, like the ones in your mojito, are a great remedy for nausea and those annoying headaches. Rubbing peppermint oil on your temples can help alleviate headaches by reducing inflammation and providing a cooling sensation to your head. Menthol, one of the active ingredients in mint, has been shown to help relax and soothe the stomach, getting rid of that tight and anxious feeling you get whenever you feel sick.

Possible Side Effects, Contraindications, and Drug Interactions

Mint is generally considered safe. If you are currently suffering from gastrointestinal reflux disease, mint may make the condition worse.

Peppermint oil in large doses can be toxic, and pure menthol is poisonous and should never, ever be taken internally.

Do not apply mint oil to the face of an infant or small child, as this can cause spasms and inhibit breathing.

Use caution with products that contain mint in those who have or have previously had gallstones.

As always, talk to your doctor or health care practitioner if any of the medications you are taking interact with mint.

Mint Care Guide

Growing mint indoors could be one of the easiest choices you make all year. Mint thrives in container gardens. Find a pot with drainage holes and buy some mint from your local gardening store to get started.

Lighting: Place in a window with indirect light, preferably an east-facing window in the spring and summer, and a south-facing window in the fall and winter.

Water: Make sure to water your plants often, keeping the soil moist. However, don't overwater, causing your soil to be soggy. Mint does not want to be overly wet. Once the soil becomes dry to the touch, watering is needed.

Soil: Use well-draining potting soil.

Temperature: Make sure the temperature remains around 65°F to 70°F. Also, mint likes humidity. Make sure to mist the leaves between watering.

Recipes and Remedies

Growing mint in your home will guarantee an abundance of opportunity for DIY activities, not to mention its popularity in a ton of amazing recipes and remedies alike. From toothpaste to deodorant, you'll feel fresh and clean with the right dose of mint.

Homemade Mint Toothpaste

Lots of toothpaste products on the shelves today include ingredients that are unpronounceable and don't belong in our bodies; that includes certain toothpastes. Making your own household products is most always the simpler, safer, and better-quality avenue.

Ingredients:

- 1 tablespoon fresh mint leaves, chopped
- ¼ cup water
- ½ teaspoon baking soda
- ½ teaspoon cornstarch
- ½ teaspoon grapeseed oil

Instructions:

1. Place your mint leaves in a pot with water and bring to a boil. Remove from the heat and let the leaves steep for twenty minutes.
2. Combine the baking soda, cornstarch, and grapeseed oil. Mix until smooth.
3. Strain the cooled mint tea and add the liquid to the baking soda mixture. Add the mixture to a pot and bring to a boil, stirring until it's slightly thick and smooth.
4. Cool completely and place in an airtight container.

Fresh Mint Tea

Forget the store-bought mint tea packs that cost you five dollars. Why not take mint leaves from your overabundant garden and make the freshest tea you've ever tasted—and the cheapest. Making mint tea is effortless and incredibly refreshing, and if it's a hot day, why not make iced mint tea?

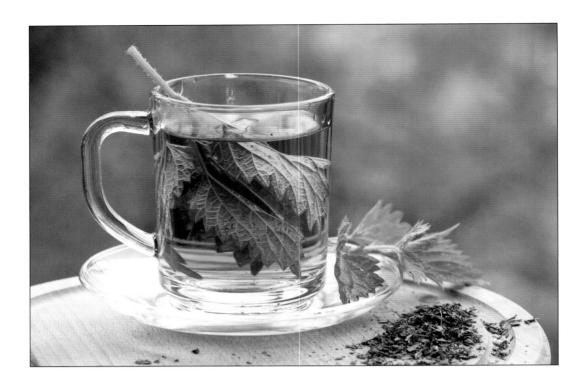

Ingredients:

- A few sprigs of fresh mint
- Water
- Honey to taste

Instructions:

1. Take your mint sprigs and place them in a pot with two cups of water.
2. Bring the pot to a boil; boil for three minutes.
3. Strain the water from the pot, and add honey to taste.

Mint Tincture

Making your own tincture from any herb is a perfect way to obtain all the health benefits of the oils. Your mint tincture can be added as a flavoring to cocktails, placed in your morning tea, added to your favorite baked goods, or even used as an insect repellent. Dampening your cotton balls with mint extract and placing them in areas where insects and pests are found can deter them from the area; just keep them away from your pets.

Placing a few drops of mint tincture to a carrier oil such as coconut oil, olive oil, or jojoba can turn your mint into an amazing salve for chest congestion, sore muscles, joint pain, and tension headaches. The list is endless when it comes to using mint, especially a mint tincture.

Ingredients:

- A bundle of fresh mint leaves
- Sealable jar, such as a mason jar
- High-proof alcohol, such as vodka
- Brown glass container

Instructions:

1. Chop or bruise your mint leaves; no need to remove the stems. You can use a mortar and pestle or simply a knife in order to expose the oils. Make sure to throw away any dark or odd-looking leaves, as they could be rotting.
2. Stuff your bundle of chopped/bruised mint leaves in a mason jar. Leave as little as a half inch at the top if you want your tincture to be stronger.
3. Once the leaves are packed inside the jar, pour in the alcohol, completely covering the mint. Close the jar tightly.
4. Let the jar sit for several weeks (three to six weeks) in a dark place; kitchen cabinets work well. If you want your tincture to be stronger, leave the jar sitting longer.

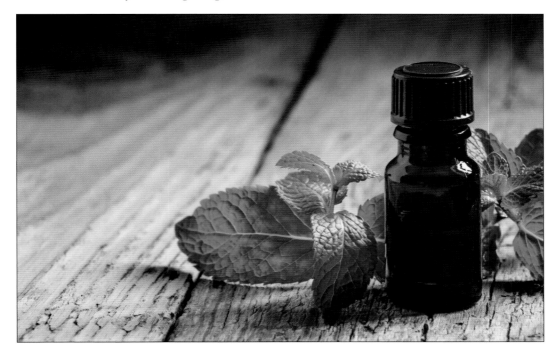

5. Shake your jar a couple of times a week to speed up the process.
6. Taste a drop of your tincture to decide if it's perfect for you.
7. When it's done, strain your liquid into a brown glass container. You can also put the liquid through a coffee filter to fully separate out the leaves and sediment.
8. Your tincture should last about six months. Use it before it goes bad!

Mint Coconut All-Natural Deodorant

More and more, people are turning towards all-natural deodorant to help hide their spicy aromas. Placing toxic ingredients on your skin means that some of it enters your bloodstream without being metabolized. While not everything you rub on your glowing skin enters your bloodstream, blood tests show that many substances commonly found in deodorant products can in fact get past the skin and enter the body. Research has also shown that some of the compounds found in deodorants are absorbed and stored in fat cells, which can react with your underarm tissue and disrupt hormones. Some researchers believe this can contribute to reproductive issues and even cancer, so when it comes to your health, choosing the most natural route is the best way to go.

Ingredients:
- 2 tablespoons coconut oil
- 2 tablespoons baking soda
- 5 drops peppermint essential oil, or your homemade mint tincture (Add more or less according to your needs.)

Instructions:
1. Melt the coconut oil to room temperature.
2. Mix together all the ingredients, stirring with a fork.
3. Place in a jar and let it sit in the fridge until it hardens.

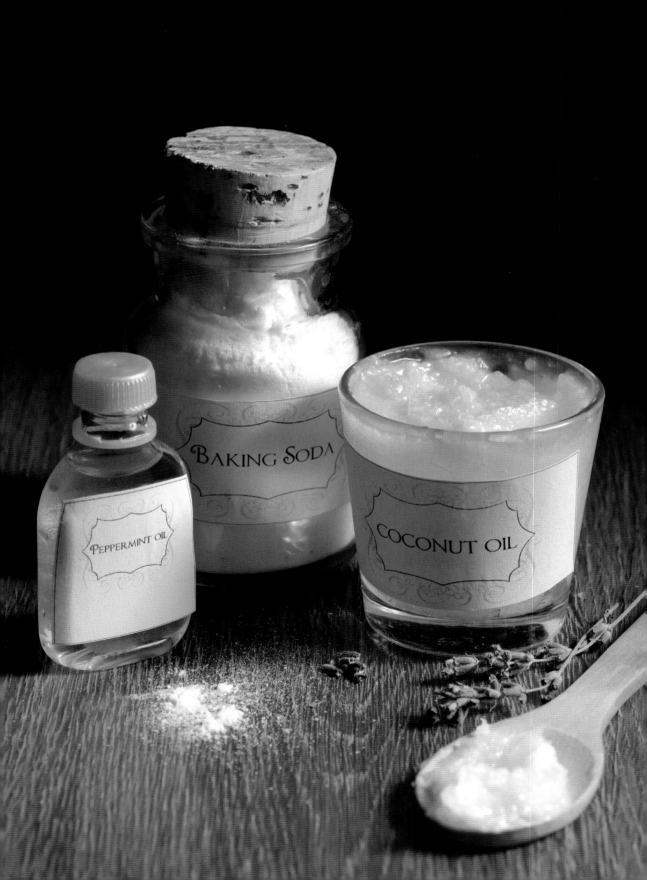

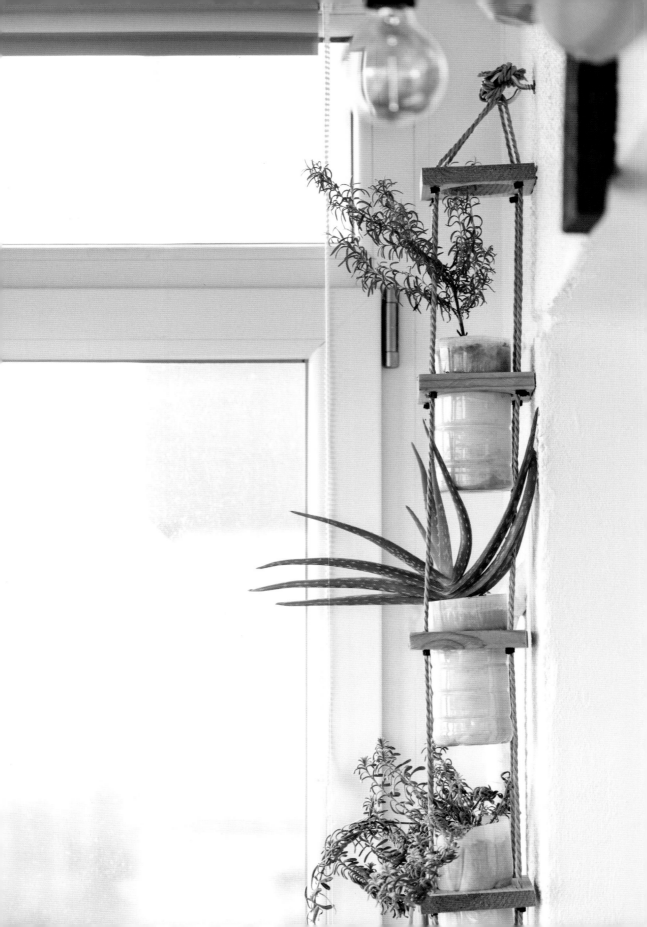

Conclusion

As we look into the future of health care, nothing will prepare us more than looking back—looking back on ancient traditions and home remedies; using the same herbs and medicinals used by our ancestors; and not taking for granted the knowledge of the doctors, shamans, herbalists, and health care workers before us.

No longer will the focus of health and wellness be on killing disease; rather, the focus will be on promoting health and preventing illness. For a majority of the illnesses and diseases out there, lifestyle is the number-one factor. According to the World Health Organization, 60 percent of related factors to individual health and quality of life are correlated with lifestyle.[76]

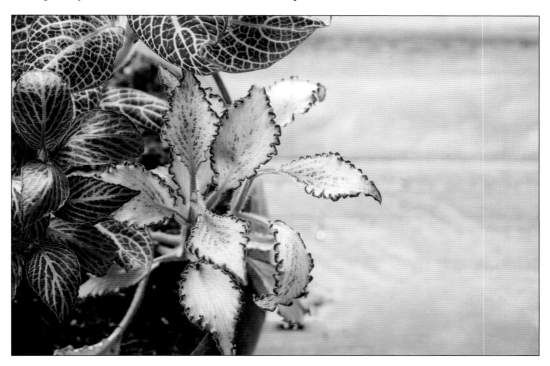

Lifestyle Matters

Lifestyle may seem like a term thrown around too often with no actual meaning behind it, but the truth of the matter is every decision you make on a daily basis affects your health and your future outcomes. Your diet, weight, sleep, exercise, sex life, medication use, drug use, stress, recreation, hobbies, fun, relationships, and more can all affect your health and well-being. And before you give up and say, "Everything is out to kill me so who cares," think about this: of course we are all going to die, but eating well and making sure you make the best choices isn't just a naive way to avoid death. Making good choices ultimately leads to a longer health span—meaning the amount of time in your life that you are healthy enough to enjoy all the activities in life that makes life worth living.

Many of us have an elderly grandparent or loved one who lived to an old age, only to suffer the last twenty years of their life with a chronic illness or disease, skeletons of their former selves.

And while we won't know for sure what eventually triggered the Alzheimer's, dementia, heart disease, cancers, chronic illness, autoimmune disorders, and more, we can attribute a major portion of it to what we eat, how we move, and so much more. Pay attention to those around you who thrive into old age, the ones who continue to have a zest for life, who keep dancing, laughing, and enjoying their time. What are they doing differently?

YOUR GENES AREN'T YOUR DESTINY

As medicine becomes further advanced, we're learning more and more about the human genome and what our own DNA says about us and our future health. And while decades ago doctors believed knowing the human genome was the solution to every disease and illness, we're learning that environment and lifestyle play

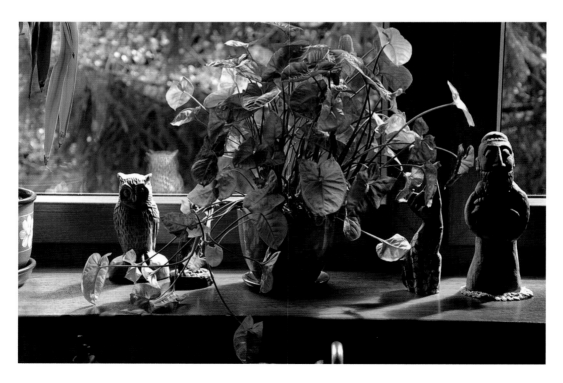

a much bigger role than anticipated. Yes, our genes matter, but they play a more passive role than expected.

THE HUMAN GENOME PROJECT

The Human Genome Project (HGP), one of the greatest feats in medical history, was also the most anticipated health project in history. This fifteen-year international collaborative research program had a goal of mapping and understanding the entire genome of human beings. Scientists believed that mapping our genomes would provide us with a cure for every disease and be the answer to all our health woes.

Because of the HGP, we know that our genome contains about 3.2 billion adenine, cytosine, guanine, and thymine bases—the molecules which make up the DNA code. We also know more about chromosomes—for example, chromosome 1 contains the most genes (3,168), while the Y chromosome contains the least (344). The list of what we learned goes on.

And while the Human Genome Project still provides the science and medical community with important and necessary information about our health and history, it also left us with a lot of questions. But most importantly, we learned the environment, from conception to the present, plays a huge role in influencing our health. As many wise people have noted, genes may load the gun, but the environment pulls the trigger.

This idea that our lifestyle and environment influence how our genes are expressed is called epigenetics. We are influenced by our environment from conception—this includes what our mother ate during pregnancy; how stressed she was; the method of birth; whether or not we were breastfed; both our mother's and father's health at the time of conception; exposure to toxins such as smoking, chemical pollutants, and infectious agents at the beginning of life; all the way to where we currently live—the climate, urban versus rural, our economic, social, and physiological influences, finances, stress, and more.

The nature-versus-nurture debate has existed for ages, and we're just now realizing that this distinction is not mutually exclusive. In fact, the two factors interact in very specific ways that alter gene behavior. The interaction of the environment with our given genetics determines the ways our genes are turned on or off, like a switch.

This is why identical twins are similar but not the same. They may have the same genetics, age, and pregestational environment, but even with diseases that have a high genetic heritability, chances are only one of them will have it. In other words, if one twin has schizophrenia, there is only a 50 percent chance the other twin will have it too.

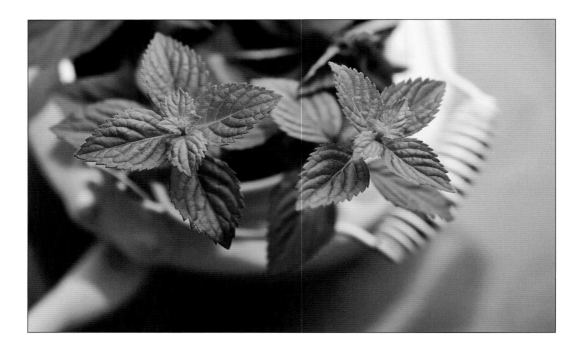

That's not to say that your inherited genetics doesn't matter—amazing information can be had from your personal genome, and that information will help you decide how to change your lifestyle to best fit your personal needs.

OVERWHELMING OPTIONS

In the end, realizing that your environment is the primary factor of health and human disease can be . . . well . . . overwhelming. With countless fitness gurus proclaiming the benefits of their patented protein bars, you may think there is no one way to health. And that's correct. There is no one way to health, and as we learn more about our personal genetics, we can begin to personally retrofit our diets and lifestyles to match our needs.

Food Matters

Until the future reaches our doorsteps, there are several things you can do to positively affect your genome and prevent illness and disease. For example, quit the fast food! How can we expect to thrive in this world while eating Twinkies and sitting on our butts all day? For all that's good and decent in our world we have to collectively change our addiction to fast food and a sedentary lifestyle.

Diet is one of the most important factors for health and wellness, and it's necessary to eat real food. This includes as much organic, local food as possible, and eating as many vegetables as possible (this doesn't include french fries; fried potatoes don't count). People like to claim they don't like vegetables, opting for hamburgers and fries, but this excuse for nutritional insufficiency is not funny when someone gets sick, hurt, or worse. Hamburgers can be a part of a healthy, well-rounded diet, but only if your diet actually consists of healthy foods.

Don't let the latest nutrition research studies or fads get you confused and nihilistic; get ahold of yourself and eat what is universally healthy. There will never be an article which declares fried foods healthy, or that you should eat dessert every morning for a well-rounded breakfast. No one will ever tell you to stop eating a wide variety of vegetables, and for all that's holy in our world, stop with the low-fat cookies and *drop* the margarine. Just eat real, whole foods. Butter, olive oil, avocados, yes!

EATING MORE DIVERSELY

Eating a diverse array of vegetables and herbs and fresh, organic offerings will provide you with the range of nutrients you need to keep your body strong and healthy. Growing your own houseplants and herbs will make it easier to incorporate the healthiest foods into your diet. From basil to broccoli sprouts, mint, rosemary, and other delicious greenery, you're helping to prevent further disease and illnesses. Not to mention, what you grow in your own home will be guaranteed organic, and local.

Make sure to eat seasonally for your region—you don't have to spend seven dollars on blueberries if it's February in Chicago—and utilize your local farmers' markets as much as you can during the warmer months. Not only are you helping yourself, but you're supporting your local farmers, who work hard to bring you organic, healthy, and delicious food.

Exercise and Move More

Moving your body to be healthy is an understatement. We live in a time where Dormant Butt Syndrome is an actual . . . syndrome! Yes, sitting on your butt too long actually causes your gluteal muscles to forget what to do, leaving you in chronic pain from your low back to your knees. No joke. If this isn't a sign of the times, I don't know what is.

Don't let your butt go dormant and start moving your body. I'm not talking about becoming an Olympian or completing a triathlon, but I am saying start walking every day. Back in my college days, I took a physical education class called Walking for Fitness to obtain my last gym credit for graduation, and of course I thought it was going to be easy as pie. Who creates a Walking for Fitness gym class in the first place? Little did I know, we'd be pumping up hills, speed walking for our lives, making sure our hearts were pounding. I almost fainted several times that semester due to my inability to believe walking to be a true sport. Little did I know, research is backing up the enormous benefits of walking.

Walking for as little as twenty minutes a day can trigger antiaging processes and repair old DNA! Yes, you read that right. Not only that, but those who take brisk thirty-minute walks daily benefit from antiaging affects that may add an additional three to seven years of life! Those people who speed walk at the mall know what's good for them!

Sleep More

If you want to lose weight, maintain your energy, boost your brain, improve memory, and decrease your likelihood of getting Alzheimer's, depression, anxiety, and other chronic illnesses, think about your sleep habits. Sleep is one of the most important indicators of health, and losing just thirty minutes of sleep per day can promote weight gain and negatively affect blood sugar control.

For those of us who have insomnia, learning about all the negative health associations with lack of sleep only makes getting a good night's rest even more difficult. But it's still necessary to call out the importance of a restful night and place importance on this necessary health aid. Getting sleep is probably the cheapest, and easiest (for some), thing you can do for your health. No health supplement can boast the same amazing benefits as sleep. From making you live longer to reducing inflammation, enhancing creativity, improving mood and memory, aid-

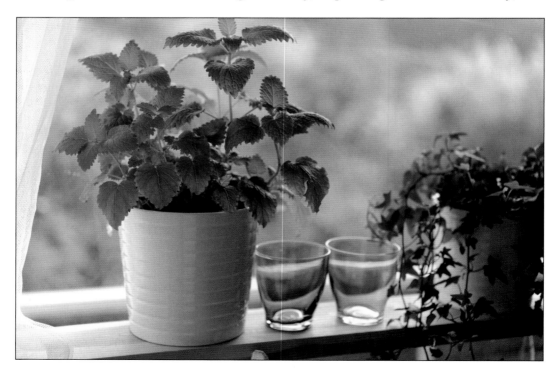

ing in weight loss, lowering stress, and more, if we don't get a good night's sleep, we're screwed.

Reduce the amount of screen time before bed; looking at your phone, iPads, laptops, and any other technological screen only prevents your body from becoming sleepy, reducing your natural hormone production of melatonin. Melatonin regulates the sleep-wake cycle, but every time you are on Facebook right before bed, your brain's activity increases, and prevents you from calming down and transitioning into a peaceful, sleepy state of mind.

Do yourself a favor and read a real book before bed; who doesn't fall asleep after five pages of *Moby Dick*? It's the perfect place to read all the classics, and if it ends up taking you five years per book, so be it. At least you're sleeping well.

Reduce Your Stress

The statistics are pretty grim. According to the American Institute of Stress, stress is the central cause of 60 percent of all human illness and disease, with three out of every four visits to the doctor being related to stress.

A landmark twenty-year study conducted by the University of London concluded that unmanaged reactions to stress were a more dangerous risk factor for cancer and heart disease than cigarette smoking.

And a study duplicated by Harvard and Stanford found that high job demands increase the odds of having an illness diagnosed by a doctor by 35 percent, with long work hours increasing the chances of early death by almost 20 percent.

Stress is making us sick, and not just sick in the head.

It's a never-ending cycle of overwork, decreased health, bad food choices, bad overall choices as a way to feel better about our other bad choices, decreased health from bad choices, increased purchases of Snickers and Pizza Hut cheesy crust pizzas, all leading to overall depression and anxiety. See what I mean? It's a never-ending cycle.

And while we are expected to work more for the same amount of money, we aren't given many breaks either. The US, unlike other industrialized nations, doesn't legally require workers to take time off. Spain and England require thirty days' vacation per year, and on average, the French take seven weeks of vacation per year. The US average is ten work days off and eight national holidays.

We're tired. And we should be jealous and a bit upset.

If we don't do something about this persistent problem, our bodies are going to rebel, and I promise you it won't be fun.

With an increase of chronic disease, we're already experiencing the consequences of our overworked lifestyle. Anxiety, depression, digestion issues, heart disease, sleep problems, weight gain, memory and cognition impairment, lousy moods, chronic pain, lowered immunity, autoimmune diseases, and poor choices at the racetrack can all be traced back to chronic stress.

But before we get all depressed and stressed out, let's take a step back and breathe. Really. Stop and relax. Finding ways to decrease the stress in your life is as important as getting a good night's rest, eating your vegetables, and moving your body. And there are many things you can do to alleviate such stress—acupuncture, herbal medicine, exercise, sauna use, meditation, vacations, reading your favorite romance novel, watching your favorite romantic comedy—ya know, anything you enjoy! With more and more technology and awareness of the importance of reducing your stress levels, it's easier today than ever to find ways to reduce your stress and maintain your mental and physical health. But you have to start making yourself a priority.

Sunlight

If you live in the Pacific Northwest, you're missing out on one of the most important health commodities out there . . . the sun and vitamin D. Vitamin D is actually a steroid hormone, of which our main source is from the big star in the sky. The sun is one of the greatest vitamins in the universe, and no matter what anyone tells you, we need that bright ball of fire for our health. Also known as the sunshine vitamin, vitamin D is fat soluble and can affect as many as two thousand genes in the body.

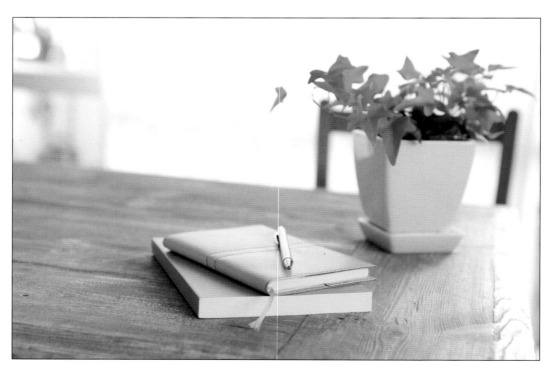

Our bodies naturally produce vitamin D when exposed to the sun, but that doesn't include when your body is slathered in a variety of sunscreens. One of the most important aspects of vitamin D is its ability to boost the immune system, important for bone growth and development, as well as providing improved resistance to a variety of diseases. And if you think calcium is the number-one preventer of bone abnormalities such as osteomalacia or osteoporosis, you're wrong! Vitamin D is more important for decreasing the risk of such disorders.

Vitamin D also reduces your risk of developing multiple sclerosis, heart disease, depression, and the flu. Have you ever wondered why flu season occurs in the fall? Because that's when people start having a decrease in their vitamin D consumption due to the decrease in daylight from summer. When we see a decrease in sunshine, we see a decrease in vitamin D, which means more susceptibility to illness. It all makes sense now!

If you live in a big city where tall buildings block the sunlight, have darker skin, spend a lot of time indoors, or live in an area with high pollution, this could all impede your ability to get vitamin D.

Making sure you get enough sunlight during the summer, and supplementing during the winter, will help you stay healthier, sunnier, and happier.

Start Small

With so much information out there, it can be a confusing mess on what to do with your health. Luckily, there is a lot you can do in your own home to become the healthiest version of yourself. Growing your own plants can be an enjoyable healthy activity, which not only lowers stress, but gives you a harvest of health for an amazing array of remedies and recipes.

Growing plants indoors is one of the easiest and most accessible ways to improve your health and wellness. Simply placing houseplants in your home will help you breathe cleaner air, improve your focus and well-being, and provide an impressive decor. Start small and expand out once you get your bearings, working your way up the plant and herbal ladder.

Becoming healthy doesn't have to be an arduous task with wake-up calls to the gym at five in the morning or depriving yourself of delicious foods. Creating repeatable habits will make you healthier, one mint leaf at a time.

Endnotes

1   Wolverton, B.C. et al., "Interior Landscape Plants for Indoor Air Pollution Abatement." NASA. July 01, 1989. https://ntrs.nasa.gov/archive/nasa/casi.ntrs.nasa.gov/19930072988.pdf.

2   Q. Li et al., "Effect of Phytoncide from Trees on Human Natural Killer Cell Function," *International Journal of Immunopathology and Pharmacology* 22, no. 4 (October 1, 2009): 951–59, https://doi.org/10.1177/039463200902200410.

3   "Stressed at Work? Put Potted Plants on Your Desk," Mail Online, June 13, 2011, http://www.dailymail.co.uk/health/article-2002499/Stressed-work-Put-pot-plants-desk.html.

4   Min-sun Lee et al., "Interaction with Indoor Plants May Reduce Psychological and Physiological Stress by Suppressing Autonomic Nervous System Activity in Young Adults: A Randomized Crossover Study," *Journal of Physiological Anthropology* 34 (April 28, 2015): 21,

5   Erin Largo-Wight et al., "Healthy Workplaces: The Effects of Nature Contact at Work on Employee Stress and Health," *Public Health Reports* 126, no. 1_suppl (May 1, 2011): 124–30, https://doi.org/10.1177/00333549111260S116.

6   Li Qi et al., "Acute Effects of Walking in Forest Environments on Cardiovascular and Metabolic Paremeters." *European Journal of Applied Physiology* no. 111 (March 23, 2011) https://doi.org/10.1007/s00421-011-1918-z.

7   "Science: You Now Have a Shorter Attention Span Than Goldfish," *Time*, May 14, 2015, time.com/3858309/attention-spans-goldfish/.

8   Ruth K. Raanaas et al., "Benefits of Indoor Plants on Attention Capacity in an Office Setting," *Journal of Environmental Psychology* 31, no. 1 (March 1, 2011): 99–105, https://doi.org/10.1016/j.jenvp.2010.11.005.

9   Tina Bringslimark, Terry Hartig, and Grete Grindal Patil, "Psychological Benefits of Indoor Plants in Workplaces: Putting Experimental Results into Context," *Hort Science* no. 3 (June, 2007): 581–587 http://hortsci.ashspublications.org/content/42/3/581.full.pdf+html.

10 Seong-Hyun Park and Richard H. Mattson, "Ornamental Indoor Plants in Hospital Rooms Enhanced Health Outcomes of Patients Recovering from Surgery," *Journal of Alternative and Complementary Medicine* 15, no. 9 (August 29, 2009): 975–80, https://doi.org/10.1089/acm.2009.0075.

11 "Flowering Plants Speed Post-Surgery Recovery," ScienceDaily, December 30, 2008, https://www.sciencedaily.com/releases/2008/12/081229104700.htm.

12 Elizabeth Landau, "From a Tree, a 'Miracle' Called Aspirin," December 22, 2010, http://www.cnn.com/2010/HEALTH/12/22/aspirin.history/index.html.

13 Ratree Maenthaisong et al., "The Efficacy of Aloe Vera Used for Burn Wound Healing: A Systematic Review," *Burns* 33, no. 6 (September 1, 2007): 713–18, https://doi.org/10.1016/j.burns.2006.10.384.

14 Rajendra Kumar Gupta et al., "Preliminary Antiplaque Efficacy of Aloe Vera Mouthwash on 4 Day Plaque Re-Growth Model: Randomized Control Trial," *Ethiopian Journal of Health Sciences* 24, no. 2 (April 2014): 139–44. https://www.ncbi.nlm.nih.gov/pmc/articles/PMC4006208/.

15 Bushra Karim et al., "Effect of Aloe Vera Mouthwash on Periodontal Health: Triple Blind Randomized Control Trial," *Oral Health and Dental Management* 13, no. 1 (March 2014): 14–19. https://www.ncbi.nlm.nih.gov/pubmed/24603910/.

16 Soyun Cho, et al., "Dietary Aloe Vera Supplementation Improves Facial Wrinkles and Elasticity and It Increases the Type I Procallagen Gene Expression in Human Skin *in vivo*," *The Annals of Dermatology* no. 21 (February 21, 2009), https://doi.org/10.5021/ad.2009.21.1.6.

17 Kanokporn Bhalang, Pasutha Thunyakitpisal, and Nuttanit Rungsirisatean, "Acemannan, a Polysaccharide Extracted from Aloe Vera, Is Effective in the Treatment of Oral Aphthous Ulceration," *Journal of Alternative and Complementary Medicine* 19, no. 5 (May 2013): 429–34, https://doi.org/10.1089/acm.2012.0164.

18 Neda Babaee et al., "Evaluation of the Therapeutic Effects of Aloe Vera Gel on Minor Recurrent Aphthous Stomatitis," *Dental Research Journal* 9, no. 4 (2012): 381–85. https://www.ncbi.nlm.nih.gov/pmc/articles/PMC3491322/.

19 Hiroko-Miyuki Mori et al., "Wound Healing Potential of Lavender Oil by Acceleration of Granulation and Wound Contraction through Induction of TGF-β in a Rat Model," *BMC Complementary and Alternative Medicine* 16 (May 26, 2016), https://doi.org/10.1186/s12906-016-1128-7.

20 H. woelk and S. Schlafke, "A Multi-center, double-blind, randomized study of the Lavender oil preparation Silexan in comparison to Lorazepam for generalized anxiety disorder," *Phytomedicine* 17 no. 2 (February, 2010): https://doi.org/10.1016/j.phymed.2009.10.006.

21 Peir Hossein Koulivant et al., "Review Article: Lavender and the Nervous System," *Evidence Based Complementary and Alternative Medicine* 2013 (March 14, 2013), http://dx.doi.org/10.1155/2013/681304.

22 American Congress of Obstetricians and Gynecologists, *2011 Women's Health Stats & Facts*, accessed January 31, 2018, https://www.acog.org/-/media/NewsRoom/MediaKit.pdf.

23 Tamaki Matsumoto, Hiroyuki Asakura, and Tatsuya Hayashi, "Does Lavender Aromatherapy Alleviate Premenstrual Emotional Symptoms?: A Randomized Crossover Trial," *BioPsychoSocial Medicine* 7 (May 31, 2013): 12, https://doi.org/10.1186/1751-0759-7-12.

24 Namni Goel, Hyungsoo Kim, and Raymund P. Lao, "An Olfactory Stimulus Modifies Nighttime Sleep in Young Men and Women," *The Journal of Biological and Medical Rhythm Research* 22, no. 5 (May, 2005): 889–904 https://doi.org/10.1080/07420520500263276.

25 Peir Hossein Koulivand, Maryam Khaleghi Ghadiri, and Ali Gorji, "Lavender and the Nervous System," *Evidence-Based Complementary and Alternative Medicine* 2013 (2013), https://doi.org/10.1155/2013/681304.

26 S. Johnson, "The Multifaceted and Widespread Pathology of Magnesium Deficiency," *Medical Hypotheses* 56, no. 2 (February 1, 2001): 163–70, https://doi.org/10.1054/mehy.2000.1133.

27 M. S. Seelig, "Consequences of Magnesium Deficiency on the Enhancement of Stress Reactions; Preventive and Therapeutic Implications (a Review)," *Journal of the American College of Nutrition* 13, no. 5 (October 1994): 429–46, https://www.ncbi.nlm.nih.gov/pubmed/7836621.

28 Mark Moss and Lorraine Oliver, "Plasma 1,8-Cineole Correlates with Cognitive Performance Following Exposure to Rosemary Essential Oil Aroma," *Therapeutic Advances in Psychopharmacology* 2, no. 3 (June 2012): 103–13, https://doi.org/10.1177/2045125312436573.

29 Andrew Pengelly et al., "Short-Term Study on the Effects of Rosemary on Cognitive Function in an Elderly Population," *Journal of Medicinal Food* 15, no. 1 (January 2012): 10–17, https://doi.org/10.1089/jmf.2011.0005.

30 Joseph Tai et al., "Antiproliferation Effect of Rosemary (Rosmarinus Officinalis) on Human Ovarian Cancer Cells in Vitro," *Phytomedicine: International Journal of Phytotherapy and Phytopharmacology* 19, no. 5 (March 15, 2012): 436–43, https://doi.org/10.1016/j.phymed.2011.12.012.

31 Chiung-Huei Peng et al., "Supercritical Fluid Extracts of Rosemary Leaves Exhibit Potent Anti-Inflammation and Anti-Tumor Effects," *Bioscience, Biotechnology, and Biochemistry* 71, no. 9 (September 2007): 2223–32, https://doi.org/10.1271/bbb.70199.

32 S. Y. Tsen, F. Ameri, and J. S. Smith, "Effects of Rosemary Extracts on the Reduction of Heterocyclic Amines in Beef Patties," *Journal of Food Science* 71, no. 8 (October 1, 2006): C469–73, https://doi.org/10.1111/j.1750-3841.2006.00149.x.

33 Yunes Panahi et al., "Rosemary Oil vs Minoxidil 2% for the Treatment of Androgenetic Alopecia: A Randomized Comparative Trial," *Skinmed* 13, no. 1 (February 2015): 15–21, https://www.ncbi.nlm.nih.gov/pubmed/25842469.

34 Kazuya Murata et al., "Promotion of Hair Growth by Rosmarinus Officinalis Leaf Extract," *Phytotherapy Research* 27, no. 2 (February 2013): 212–17, https://doi.org/10.1002/ptr.4712.

35 Hay IC, Jamieson M, Ormerod AD, "Randomized Trial of Aromatherapy. Successful Treatment for Alopecia Areata," *Archives of Dermatology*, 134, no. 11 (November, 1998): 1348–1352, https://www.ncbi.nlm.nih.gov/pubmed/9828867.

36 Daniel Arango et al., "Molecular Basis for the Action of a Dietary Flavonoid Revealed by the Comprehensive Identification of Apigenin Human Targets," *Proceedings of the National Academy of Sciences* 110, no. 24 (June 11, 2013): E2153–62, https://doi.org/10.1073/pnas.1303726110.

37 Janmejai K. Srivastava and Sanjay Gupta, "Antiproliferative and Apoptotic Effects of Chamomile Extract in Various Human Cancer Cells," *Journal of Agricultural and Food Chemistry* 55, no. 23 (November 1, 2007): 9470–78, https://doi.org/10.1021/jf071953k.

38 M. G. L. Hertog et al., "Dietary Antioxidant Flavonoids and Risk of Coronary Heart Disease: The Zutphen Elderly Study," *The Lancet* 342, no. 8878 (October 23, 1993): 1007–11, https://doi.org/10.1016/0140–6736(93)92876-U.

39 Janmejai K. Sirvastava, Eswar Shankar, and Sanjay Gupta, "Chamomile: A herbal medicine of the past with a bright future (Review), *Molecular Medicine Reports* 3, no. 6 (September 27, 2010): 895–901, https://doi.org/10.3892/mmr.2010.377

40 Jay D. Amsterdam et al., "A Randomized, Double-Blind, Placebo-Controlled Trial of Oral Matricaria Recutita (Chamomile) Extract Therapy of Generalized Anxiety Disorder," *Journal of Clinical Psychopharmacology* 29, no. 4 (August 2009): 378–82, https://doi.org/10.1097/JCP.0b013e3181ac935c.

41 American Heart Association. "Eating citrus fruit may lower women's stroke risk." ScienceDaily. www.sciencedaily.com/releases/2012/02/120223182638.htm (accessed February 13, 2018).

42 Maeve C. Cosgrove et al., "Dietary Nutrient Intakes and Skin-Aging Appearance among Middle-Aged American Women," *American Journal of Clinical Nutrition* 86, no. 4 (October 1, 2007): 1225–31, https://doi.org/10.1093/ajcn/86.4.1225.

43 Abdolali Mohagheghzadeh et al., "Medicinal Smokes," *Journal of Ethnopharmacology* 108, no. 2 (November 24, 2006): 161–84, https://doi.org/10.1016/j.jep.2006.09.005.

44 Chandra Shekhar Nautiyal, Puneet Singh Chauhan, and Yeshwant Laxman Nene, "Medicinal Smoke Reduces Airborne Bacteria," *Journal of Ethnopharmacology* 114, no. 3 (December 3, 2007): 446–51, https://doi.org/10.1016/j.jep.2007.08.038.

45 N. T. J. Tildesley et al., "*Salvia lavandulaefolia* (Spanish Sage) Enhances Memory in Healthy Young Volunteers," *Pharmacology, Biochemistry, and Behavior* 75, no. 3 (June 2003): 669–74, https://www.ncbi.nlm.nih.gov/pubmed/12895685.

46 "A Sage Discovery: Plant-Derived Compounds Have Potent Anti-Inflammatory Effects," ScienceDaily, July 27, 2016, https://www.sciencedaily.com/releases/2016/07/160727194408.htm.

47 Carla M. Sá et al., "Sage Tea Drinking Improves Lipid Profile and Antioxidant Defences in Humans," *International Journal of Molecular Science* 10, no. 9 (2009): 3937–3950, https://www.ncbi.nlm.nih.gov/pmc/articles/PMC2769154/.

48 Maryam Eidi, Akram Eidi, and Hamidreza Zamanizadeh, "Effect of Salvia officinalis L. leaves on serum glucose and insulin in healthy and streptozotocin-induced diabetic rats," *Journal of Ethopharmacology* 100, no. 3 (September 14, 2005): 310–313 https://doi.org/10.1016/j.jep.2005.03.008

49 S. Bommer, P. Klein, and A. Suter, "First time proof of Sage's tolerability and efficacy in menopausal women with hot flushes," *Advances in Therapy,* 28, no. 6 (June, 2011): 490–500, https://www.ncbi.nlm.nih.gov/pubmed/21630133.

50 Sammy Selim, "Antimicrobial Activity of Essential Oils against Vancomycin-Resistant Enterococci (Vre) And Escherichia Coli 0157:H7 in Feta Soft Cheese And Minced Beef Meat," *Brazilian Journal of Microbiology* 42, no. 1 (2011): 187–196, https://www.ncbi.nlm.nih.gov/pmc/articles/PMC3768948/.

51 S. J. Chatterjee et al., "The Efficacy of Dandelion Root Extract in Inducing Apoptosis in Drug-Resistant Human Melanoma Cells," *Evidence-Based Complementary and Alternative Medicine* 2011 (2011): 129045, https://doi.org/10.1155/2011/129045.

52 "Calendula," University of Maryland Medical Center, last reviewed on June 22, 2015, https://www.umm.edu/health/medical/altmed/herb/calendula.

53 "Calendula Oil," Centerchem Inc., accessed January 31, 2018, http://www.centerchem.com/Products/DownloadFile.aspx?FileID=6565.

54 "39 Proven Health Benefits of Sulforaphane (and Broccoli Sprouts)," *Selfhacked* (blog), updated October 24, 2017, https://www.selfhacked.com/blog/panacea-benefits-broccoli-sprouts-sulforaphane/.

55 Annika S. Axelsson et al., "Sulforaphane Reduces Hepatic Glucose Production and Improves Glucose Control in Patients with Type 2 Diabetes," *Science Translational Medicine* 9, no. 394 (June 14, 2017): eaah4477, https://doi.org/10.1126/scitranslmed.aah4477.

56 Charlotte N. Armah et al., "Diet rich in high glucoraphanin broccoli reduces plasma LDL cholesterol: Evidence from randomized controlled trials," *Molecular Nutrition Food Research* 59, no. 5 (May 2015): 918–926, https://www.ncbi.nlm.nih.gov/pmc/articles/PMC4692095/

57 Yang Bai et al., "Sulforaphane Protects against Cardiovascular Disease via Nrf2 Activation," *Oxidative Medicine and Cellular Longevity* 2015 (2015): 407580, https://doi.org/10.1155/2015/407580.

58 Xueqi Qu et al., "Sulforaphane Epigenetically Regulates Innate Immune Responses of Porcine Monocyte-Derived Dendritic Cells Induced with Lipopolysaccharide," *PLoS ONE* 10, no. 3 (March 20, 2015), https://doi.org/10.1371/journal.pone.0121574.

59 Jed W. Fahey et al., "Sulforaphane Inhibits Extracellular, Intracellular, and Antibiotic-Resistant Strains of *Helicobacter pylori* and Prevents BenzoPyrene-Induced Stomach Tumors," *Proceedings of the National Academy of Sciences* 99, no. 11 (May 28, 2002): 7610–15, https://doi.org/10.1073/pnas.112203099.

60 Noelle L. Johansson, Charles S. Pavia, and Jen Wei Chiao, "Growth Inhibition of a Spectrum of Bacterial and Fungal Pathogens by Sulforaphane, an Isothiocynate Product Found in Broccoli and Other Cruciferous Vegetables," *Planta Medica* 74, no. 7 (2008): 747–750, https://www.ncbi.nlm.nih.gov/pubmed/18484523.

61 Paul Talalay et al., "Sulforaphane Mobilizes Cellular Defenses That Protect Skin against Damage by UV Radiation," *Proceedings of the National Academy of Sciences of the United States of America* 104, no. 44 (October 30, 2007): 17500–505, https://doi.org/10.1073/pnas.0708710104.

62 Ji-Chun Zhang et al., "Prophylactic Effects of Sulforaphane on Depression-like Behavior and Dendritic Changes in Mice after Inflammation," *Journal of Nutritional Biochemistry* 39 (January 2017): 134–44, https://doi.org/10.1016/j.jnutbio.2016.10.004.

63 Pramod K. Dash et al., "Sulforaphane Improves Cognitive Function Administered Following Traumatic Brain Injury," *Neuroscience Letters* 460, no. 2 (August 28, 2009): 103–7, https://doi.org/10.1016/j.neulet.2009.04.028.

64 Andrea Tarozzi et al., "Sulforaphane as a Potential Protective Phytochemical against Neurodegenerative Diseases," *Oxidative Medicine and Cellular Longevity* 2013 (2013), https://doi.org/10.1155/2013/415078.

65 Jingzhu Zhang et al., "Beneficial Effects of Sulforaphane Treatment in Alzheimer's Disease May Be Mediated through Reduced HDAC1/3 and Increased P75NTR Expression," *Frontiers in Aging Neuroscience* 9 (May 1, 2017), https://doi.org/10.3389/fnagi.2017.00121.

66 Kanwaljit Singh et al., "Sulforaphane Treatment of Autism Spectrum Disorder (ASD)," *Proceedings of the National Academy of Sciences of the United States of America* 111, no. 43 (October 28, 2014): 15550–55, https://doi.org/10.1073/pnas.1416940111.

67 Richard Zhou, Jianjun Lin, and Defeng Wu, "Sulforaphane Induces Nrf2 and Protects Against CYP2E1-Dependent Binge Alcohol–Induced Liver Steatosis,"

Biochimica et Biophysica Acta 1840, no. 1 (January 2014), https://doi.org/10.1016/j.bbagen.2013.09.018.

68 Hongxian Chen et al., "Protective Effects of the Antioxidant Sulforaphane on Behavioral Changes and Neurotoxicity in Mice after the Administration of Methamphetamine," *Psychopharmacology* 222, no. 1 (July 2012): 37–45, https://doi.org/10.1007/s00213-011-2619-3.

69 Masahiro Kikuchi et al., "Sulforaphane-Rich Broccoli Sprout Extract Improves Hepatic Abnormalities in Male Subjects," *World Journal of Gastroenterology* 21, no. 43 (November 21, 2015): 12457–67, https://doi.org/10.3748/wjg.v21.i43.12457.

70 Masahiro Kikuchi et al., "Sulforaphane-Rich Broccoli Sprout Extract Improves Hepatic Abnormalities in Male Subjects," *World Journal of Gastroenterology* 21, no. 43 (November 21, 2015): 12457–67, https://doi.org/10.3748/wjg.v21.i43.12457.

71 Jung-Ran Noh et al., "Sulforaphane Protects against Acetaminophen-Induced Hepatotoxicity," *Food and Chemical Toxicology* 80 (June 2015): 193–200, https://doi.org/10.1016/j.fct.2015.03.020.

72 Rabab H. Sayed et al., "Sulforaphane Increases the Survival Rate in Rats with Fulminant Hepatic Failure Induced by D-Galactosamine and Lipopolysaccharide," *Nutrition Research* 34, no. 11 (November 2014): 982–89, https://doi.org/10.1016/j.nutres.2014.10.003.

73 Thomas W. Kensler et al., "Modulation of the Metabolism of Airborne Pollutants by Glucoraphanin-Rich and Sulforaphane-Rich Broccoli Sprout Beverages in Qidong, China," *Carcinogenesis* 33, no. 1 (January 2012): 101–7, https://doi.org/10.1093/carcin/bgr229.

74 Avinash M. Topè and Phyllis F. Rogers, "Evaluation of Protective Effects of Sulforaphane on DNA Damage Caused by Exposure to Low Levels of Pesticide Mixture Using Comet Assay," *Journal of Environmental Science and Health, Part B, Pesticides, Food Contaminants, and Agricultural Wastes* 44, no. 7 (September 2009): 657–62, https://doi.org/10.1080/03601230903163624.

75 Jun Ho Park et al., "Sulforaphane Inhibits the Th2 Immune Response in Ovalbumin-Induced Asthma," *BMB Reports* 45, no. 5 (May 2012): 311–16, https://www.ncbi.nlm.nih.gov/pubmed/22617456.

76 E. Ziglio, C. Currie, VB. Rasmussen, "The WHO cross-national study of health behavior in school aged children from 35 countries: findings from 2001–2002," *Journal of School Health,* 74, no. 6 (August, 2004): 204–206 https://www.ncbi.nlm.nih.gov/pubmed/15468523.

About the Author

Michelle Polk is a licensed acupuncturist and board-certified herbalist who currently runs her own practice in Chicago and specializes in nutrition and herbal medicine. She also runs a blog called *Houseplant Girl* as an effort to educate and illuminate the public on the health benefits of houseplants and herbs, as well as increase confidence in people's gardening skills. From gardening to nutrition, health shouldn't be an impossible task, and it's Michelle's mission to make sure living healthy is within reach.

Index

lemons and, 81
   sage and, 91
antiviral properties
   aloe vera and, 40
   broccoli sprouts and, 121
   calendula and, 111
anxiety. *see also* stress
   broccoli sprouts and, 121
   chamomile used for reducing, 75, 78
   lavender used for, 54, 56
aphrodisiac, 51, 109
apigenin, 74
aplastic anemia, 7
apoptosis, 74
artemisinin, 22
arthritis, 74, 82
aspirin, 21–22, 76
Asteraceae/Compositae family, 73
asthma, 76, 81, 91, 94, 123
Ativan, 54, 57
attention span, 13–14
autism, 122
Ayurveda, 99

B
B6 vitamins, 40, 66, 82
bacteria, burning medicinal herbs and
   clearing the air of, 90–91. *see also*
   antibacterial properties
baldness, rosemary and, 67–68
bamboo palm, 11
barbituates, 76
bath salts, lavender, 62–63
Bayer, 22
B-complex vitamins, 99
bee balm, 95
beeswax
   in calendula lip balm, 114–115
   for lavender balm, 60, 62
benzene, 6, 7, 9, 10, 11
benzodiazepines, 57, 76
beta-carotene, 110
Bioscience, Biotechnology, and Biochemistry,
   67
bleeding
   chamomile and risk of, 76
   sage used to stop, 89
blood pressure
   broccoli sprouts and, 120, 124
   chamomile, 76

dandelions and, 100
   rosemary and, 68
blood sugar
   aloe vera and, 43
   chamomile and, 76
   dandelion and, 100, 101
   rosemary and, 68
   sage and, 94
blood thinning drugs, 68, 76, 103
Bo He, 129
boils, 26, 99
bone health, dandelions and, 100–101
boston fern, 9
Brassica oleracea. See broccoli sprouts
Brault, Robert, 1
Brazilian Journal of Microbiology, 96
breast cancer, 74, 120
breastfeeding
   broccoli sprouts and, 124
   calendula and, 111
   lavender and, 57
   mint and, 131
   rosemary and, 68
Broccoli Sprout Dip, 127
broccoli sprouts, 117–127
   Broccoli Sprout Dip, 127
   growing/care of, 124–125
   health benefits of, 117, 118–123
   Longevity Broccoli Smoothie, 125–126
   maximizing SFN in, 125
   recommended daily intake of, 125
   side effects and drug interactions with,
      123–124
Bugg, Jim, 1
Burbank, Luther, 35
burns
   aloe vera and, 41, 48–49
   lavender and, 52
   sunburn, 39, 121
butter, sage, 97

C
calcium, 40, 65, 82, 91, 99, 100
calcium oxalate crystals, 10–11
calendula, 109–115
   Calendula Facial Toner, 114
   Calendula Lip Balm, 114–115
   Calendula Tea for Urinary Tract
      Infections, 113
   growing and care of, 112

sodium, 40, 100
soil
    for calendula, 112
    for dandelion, 103
    for lavender plant, 58
    for lemon trees, 85
    for mint plant, 132
    for rosemary plant, 69
    for sage plant, 94
sore throats, 24, 89, 110, 113, 131
spider plant, 10
sprouts. *See* broccoli sprouts
staph bacteria, 26–27
staphlococcus aureus, 26
stomach pain/ache
    chamomile for, 75
Streptococcus mutans, 41–42
stress
    chamomile flower tea for, 78
    hospital plants and, 17
    importance of managing, 145–146
    lavender used to treat, 54, 57, 62
    plants lowering, 11–14
    rosemary used for reducing, 68
substance abuse, 122
succulent family, 37
sulforaphane (SFN), 117, 118, 120–122,
    123, 125
sunburn, 39, 121
sunflower family, 100
sunlight, 146–147
sustainability, 28
sweetgrass, 95
sweet wormwood, 22
sympathetic nervous system, 13

T
Taraxacum. See dandelion plant
Taxol, 22
teas
    calendula, 113
    Dandelion Root, 104
    mint, 133–134
    rosemary digestive, 71
tea tree oil
    aloe vera hand sanitizer, 47–48
    used with lavender, 53
technology, 3–4, 14–15
temperature
    for growing lavender plant, 58

    for growing lemon trees, 85
    for growing mint, 133
    for growing sage plant, 94
Therapeutic Advances in
    Psychpharmacology, 66–67
thujone, 93
thyme, 68, 95
tinctures
    mint, 134–136
    sleepy time chamomile, 77–78
toothpaste, mint, 133
toxicity
    Chinese evergreen and, 10
    deodorant products and, 136
    lavender oil and, 57
    Peace Lily plant and, 10
    peppermint oil and, 132
    rosemary oil and, 68
    sage essential oil and, 94
toxic pollutants inside the home, 5
traditional Chinese medicine, ix, vii
    dandelion used in, 99, 101
    mint and, 129
    use of sage in, 92
trichloroethylene, 6, 9, 10, 11
troubleshooting aloe vera plant, 43–44
turkey tail, 21
turmeric, 33
Tu, Youyou, 22
twins, 141

U
ulcerative colitis, 39, 68
ulcers, 68, 89, 110, 111, 123
University of London, 145
University of Pennsylvania, 75
University of Windsor, Canada, 102
Uppsala University, 13
Uppsala University, Sweden, 13
urinary tract infections, 102, 113
UVA radiation, 121
uva-ursi, 102

V
Valium, 57
vitamin A, 91, 100, 104, 110
vitamin B6, 64–65, 82
vitamin C, 82, 83, 85, 91, 99, 117
Vitamin D, 146–147
vitamin E, 91, 110

vitamin E oil
  aloe burn cream, 48
  aloe vera hand sanitizer, 47–48
  calendula lip balm, 114–115
  lavender balm, 60, 62
  lavender bath salts, 62–63
vitamin K, 91, 100–101, 104
vitamin K1, 117
vitamins and minerals
  in aloe vera, 40
  in dandelion, 99, 100
  in lemons, 82
  in rosemary, 65–66
  in sage, 91
vodka
  aloe vera hand sanitizer, 47–48
  mint tincture, 135
  for sleepy time chamomile tincture, 77–78

W
walking, health benefits of, 143–144
Warfarin, 68, 76
watering
  aloe vera plant, 43
  calendula, 112
  chamomile, 77
  dandelion, 103
  lavender, 58

mint, 132
rosemary, 69
sage, 94
Wesleyan University, 56
West Nile virus, 28
white sage, burning, 94
willow bark, 22
wine, dandelion, 105–106
witch hazel, in DIY Chamomile Skin
  Toner, 79
workplace, plants in, 13, 15
World Health Organization (WHO), 7, 13, 23
wormwood, 21
wounds, healing
  with calendula, 110, 111
  with lavender, 53

X
Xanax, 57
xylene, 6, 9, 10, 11

Y
yarrow, 95, 102
ylang-ylang, 46–47

Z
zinc, 99